# TERROR HIGHWAY 193

Also by Susan Freire-Korn:

*Soul Sisters, Come onto My House*, discussion on cultural sensitivity and human kindness

*We the People … The Best of the Best*, how to reach your fullest potential in corporate America

*The Brown Rabbit … Let the Truth Be Told*, a.k.a. Kate Virginia, an inspiring book about domestic violence and child abuse

# TERROR HIGHWAY

## A GUIDE FOR THE SUDDENLY DISABLED

SUSAN FREIRE-KORN, MSHSA

iUniverse, Inc.
Bloomington

**Terror Highway 193**
**A Guide for the Suddenly Disabled**

The information, ideas, and suggestions in this book are not intended as a substitute for professional medical advice. Before following any suggestions contained in this book, you should consult your personal physician. Neither the author nor the publisher shall be liable or responsible for any loss or damage allegedly arising as a consequence of your use or application of any information or suggestions in this book.

iUniverse books may be ordered through booksellers or by contacting:

iUniverse
1663 Liberty Drive
Bloomington, IN 47403
www.iuniverse.com
1-800-Authors (1-800-288-4677)

Because of the dynamic nature of the Internet, any web addresses or links contained in this book may have changed since publication and may no longer be valid. The views expressed in this work are solely those of the author and do not necessarily reflect the views of the publisher, and the publisher hereby disclaims any responsibility for them.

Any people depicted in stock imagery provided by Thinkstock are models, and such images are being used for illustrative purposes only.

Certain stock imagery © Thinkstock.

ISBN: 978-1-4759-3934-7 (sc)
ISBN: 978-1-4759-3933-0 (hc)
ISBN: 978-1-4759-3932-3 (e)

Library of Congress Control Number: 2012912913

Printed in the United States of America

iUniverse rev. date: 07/26/2012

This book is dedicated to my husband, Jean-Pierre Korn. He made a split-second decision to "take the hit" for me in the head-on car accident in which we were involved in 2009. If he had not, I may not be here today and for certain would have lost my left arm. I have never known a man who would go the extra mile for me, let alone risk his life for me. I will be eternally grateful that he made the choice to spare my life. I love you, my dear husband, and you are the love of my life.

# CONTENTS

# PREFACE

After having a head-on collision and surviving it, I wanted to share my experiences in order to help others. By telling the story of my journey, I hope to assist both the suddenly disabled person and his or her care provider on the road to recovery, informing them about what to expect during the healing and recovery process, the value of following a physician's advice, and the importance of listening to the physical therapists who offer many ways to help people heal and become whole again.

The helpful guide in the back of this book provides a full explanation of the value of a quality hospital, rehabilitation center, and home care service. It talks about selecting the right medical doctor for you and offers helpful hints for regaining your independence. It will inspire you to progress from using a wheelchair, a walker, crutches, or a cane to being whole again in spirit, body, and mind.

If you are a care provider, family member, or dear friend of someone who is rehabilitating from an sudden disability, this book will educate you and help you understand what the patient's needs are and the emotional turmoil he or she experiences when surviving an injury, an accident, or a horrific event. It is also a helpful guide for the care provider to understand the day-to-day process of the healing and recovery period.

The book explains the value of family and friends, what one may need when moving back home again, and what to expect in the unexpected. It gives advice for when there are additional surgeries and offers positive-thinking methods to eliminate flashbacks and negative thoughts. It also includes a discussion on post-traumatic stress disorder in order to help others understand and identify the process the patient must endure to move forward in the healing and recovery period. In addition, there are checklists of activities for the homebound, ideas for celebrating your gains and accomplishments, and better-lifestyle hints for the suddenly disabled.

# Acknowledgments

I would like to acknowledge the men and women of the first-response teams, the physicians, surgeons, and physical therapists who make a difference in the lives of others in need of their skills, talents, and services. I would also like to thank the first person, a lovely young lady named Danielle, who took the first step to reach out to me and ask if I had a cell phone to call a family member and let him or her know what had happened. My husband and I will be forever in debt to these caring individuals.

The fire departments' first-response rescue teams risked their lives speeding in a thick fog to save our lives. The emergency helicopter could not save us because of unsafe weather conditions; however, the Georgetown Fire Department and the Cool Fire Department came to our rescue. They freed us by using the Jaws of Life on our mangled truck. They are responsible for my husband being alive today because they administered advanced life support to him once in the ambulance and kept him alive until we reached the trauma center thirty-eight miles away in Roseville, California. Thank you for risking your lives every day to help save others in need.

# INTRODUCTION

I wrote this book to share my experiences of surviving a head-on collision. My recovery process covers three years of enduring four surgeries and extensive physical therapy sessions. My journey through the recovery process found me in two hospitals and one rehabilitation center (skilled nursing facility) way before my time. Through the recovery and healing process, I began to realize that my journey and experiences could be helpful to others whose lives have been turned upside down and inside out through an sudden disability. Unless you have experienced a sudden disability, it is difficult to understand the tremendous suffering, emotional turmoil, and loss of independence one endures. Hopefully this book will be instrumental in inspiring others to regain their independence, motivating them on their road to recovery.

I often thought about writing a book on disabilities due to my multiple accidents, usually falling, which I now call a "fall risk," and the many surgeries I had as a result. On separate occasions, I broke my left arm in multiple places, broke my right leg in two places, had my left leg crushed by a truck, twisted both ankles, and tore my right knee. I have had emergency surgeries from a bursting appendix and gall bladder problems, and an exploratory laparotomy at one in the morning for an abdominal pregnancy. These injuries and surgeries plus others led me to believe I knew all about the healing and recovery process and had enough experience and knowledge to write about the topic of sudden disabilities, but I was wrong.

Experts say that most accidents happen in your home or very close to your home. We were less than one mile away from our home when the accident occurred. Nothing could have prepared me for the events of January 2, 2009, that would lead me to realize I knew very little about bodily injuries and disabilities. The results of this accident left one person dead on impact, my husband in the "valley of death" fighting for his life, and me with one arm for two years. Here is the story of our journey on the long road to healing and recovery.

# PART I:

# THE ACCIDENT THAT CHANGED OUR LIVES FOREVER

The town of Cool, California, is on Route 49 between Auburn and Placerville on a hill at an elevation of more than 1,500 feet (450 meters). It is in an area full of trees, horse and hiking trails, camping spots, and other recreational activities. It's located in the Sierra Nevada Foothills about thirty-eight miles from Roseville, California, and approximately one hundred miles from Reno, Nevada.

My husband, Jean-Pierre, and I live in Cool, just ten miles from where gold was discovered in Coloma, California. In the summer, we go swimming, and in the winter, we warm ourselves by the fire. Occasionally it snows—two or three times each year—just enough to look like we had a dusting of powdered sugar on the trees and ground. All year long, we enjoy the birds that come to either swim in our pond or enjoy the bird seed I supply on our back patio. I had never lived where I could enjoy a bird show right from the seat of my armchair. Each year, the Canadian snow geese fly overhead honking and then land in our pond for a swim. One winter, I discovered a group of sandhill cranes drying themselves off on our property. I could not believe the size of the beautiful birds and their wingspan.

Most days, the blue jays, chickadees, doves, finches, red-winged blackbirds, and quail visit our property for water and food. We have seen deer, foxes, rabbits, turkeys, red-tailed hawks, and coyotes from our back patios. They are truly gorgeous in their own environment.

The beautiful town of Cool straddles both Highway 193 and Highway 49. The air is fresh and free of smog, and the water is clear from our well and free of chemicals. Life here has minimal to no crime activity, and we attend the Catholic church of St. James in Georgetown, California. Life here is good to us, and we have grown to love the people and the community. When the Holiday Market moved in and Wells Fargo Bank arrived, I knew I was set for life. Then Autumn Moon Salon opened, and that is where I go for my hair coloring and pedicures. Being retired for three years, I was happy and realized my life was complete. Nothing could prepare us for the day a bomb went off in our laps and changed our lives forever.

*You gain strength, courage, and confidence by every experience in which you look fear in the face. You must do the thing you think you cannot do.*
—Eleanor Roosevelt

**What I Remember: Shock, Fear, and Pain**
I was just four days from my scheduled foot surgery. The surgeon had informed me the surgery would keep me in bed for a significant amount of time and that it would be a one-year recovery time. It was winter, and we had just returned from a trip to Reno, Nevada, as we always did every year to celebrate the

New Year. It was a particularly good year to celebrate, and we had taken my brother Anthony with us to show him how to ring in the New Year, the way we had done so for the past thirty years. This included driving to Reno, going to the delicious buffets, gambling to try our luck out at the tables, and of course shopping for all the sales after New Year's Day. Reno was a great place to do winter shopping and plan for all the future birthday gifts for our large family throughout the coming year.

It was Friday, January 2, 2009, when I could not get out of my mind that I just had not done enough partying and having fun away from my home to be settled in for a year in recovery. Due to the planned surgery on an arthritic toe that could no longer be ignored because of significant pain while walking, I was just days away from being in bed, in pain, and with my foot propped up on a stack of pillows, asking for ice packs and reaching for pain pills. I knew this scenario well enough because this was my second surgery after twelve years on the same toe. I just wanted to squeeze a little more fun out of my life before going under the knife.

I asked my husband if we could go see a cute movie called *Marley and Me* about a yellow lab. We have a yellow lab named Togo, and I was thinking it would be a lighthearted movie, and we could have some popcorn and munch out. Jean-Pierre was more than willing to grant me my last wish before facing surgery. We got up from the sofa and got ready to leave for the movie, which was scheduled for a 5:20 showing.

It was about 4:30 p.m. when we went out the door. As we left our driveway, there were no signs of severe fog. It was not until we entered Highway 193 about a half mile from our home that I noticed the fog was extremely thick. I mentioned to Jean-Pierre that maybe we should not go since it was so foggy.

I had driven in fog like this before while living in Daly City, California, and on trips driving through Fresno, but never before had I experienced it in our little town of Cool. Fog was one of my greatest fears because I had seen the terrible accidents it could cause. Just when I said, "Maybe we should turn back," I saw an oncoming car with the headlights on coming fast in our direction. It was in our lane and rushing toward us. I must have glanced away from the road because before I knew it, the car's headlights were lined up with ours. It was inevitable that we were on the course of destruction.

There was no time to yell, "Watch out!" or "I love you!" because we immediately collided in a crash of significant magnitude. My only thought in that split second was, *Well, let's see if I survive this.*

It reminds me of a 2003 movie called *End of an Affair.* The male actor explains what shock feels like and describes his lack of feelings after being "bombed" from his staircase in London, England, during World War II: "I never heard the bang. I awoke in five minutes or five seconds to a changed world. I didn't feel love, hate, jealously, and it all felt like happiness and without any pain." It was as if we had experienced a bomb going off right in the front seat of our truck.

The only difference is I heard the bang of our 1995 green GMC Sierra truck and the other driver's car, a Lexus, as we hit on impact. It was like a flash of lightning, in the time span of a flick of an eyelash, and our lives changed forever. Jean-Pierre was driving and had made a spilt-second decision to take the brunt of the impact. At the moment of impact, I knew instinctively that the driver in the other car was dead from our head-on collision. I wanted to get out of my truck and offer help, but I was unable to reach for my seatbelt to release it. I also knew Jean-Pierre was in deep trouble. My mind would not allow me to think that he could be dying right there next to me. I was not ready to let him go. He was gasping for air, and with each breath that he struggled to take, he asked me if

I was okay. He kept asking me that question until I realized I had to give him enough information to settle him down. It seemed like no matter what I said, he continued to ask me if I was okay.

I thought, *He must be in shock and panicking.* I could see him only from the corner of my eye. I knew the left side of my body was badly damaged, and it seemed like it was mostly my left arm. I kept trying to reassure Jean-Pierre that I was okay but then finally gave in and said, "It's my arm. I hurt it, and I think I broke it." I knew the damage was much worse than that, but I did not want to agitate him since he was in so much pain and trying desperately to breathe. He was literally drowning in his own blood! With each breath he took, there was a horrific gurgling sound coming from him, and I knew he was desperately trying to stay awake and alive. My mind refused to accept the fact that he could die before my eyes and I would witness his death.

Time stood still for us, and I began to worry about someone hitting us from behind. The fog was so severe, and it was a Friday evening; commuters would be driving like mad to get home.

It seemed like hours before anyone came to offer us any assistance. I knew from the impact that we were trapped in our truck, but I did not know the severity of it. Our green truck with a "winch and rack" place in the front of the truck had spared our lives. As we both sat there helplessly, I could feel my left arm floating above my head as if a balloon was attached to it and it was in midair with a feeling of weightlessness. When I tried with my right arm to bring my left arm down from floating in the air, I realized that my left arm was still at my side and not floating above my head. This sensation repeated itself several times, and each time it felt so real that I attempted with my right arm to reach up and bring my left arm back into place, only to discover it was already by my side. I had no explanation as to what was happening but just seemed to accept it.

## First Person to Come to Our Aid

God bless the people who take time from their own lives to help out others they do not know in time of trauma and despair. I understood that someone cared enough to get out of their car and come to my window when I heard a woman's soft voice speaking calmly and gently. I had lowered my window immediately after the crash because I had heard somewhere that when there is an accident to immediately open the window before the electricity fails. This very kind woman asked me if I had a cell phone. I answered yes, and she asked me if I could reach it. Again I said yes and went for my purse, which was on the floor between my legs in front of me. Without asking any questions, I was behaving like a robot, taking instructions. I handed the lady my purse. I did not look at her, so I cannot describe what she looked like. I was only in touch with her voice and instructions. I told her the cell phone was in the side pocket. She asked me who she should call. I said Charles. He is our nephew and lives about ten minutes away from us. She called him and informed him of the accident. He had mentioned he was not home and away on business but that he would notify the rest of his family. Jean-Pierre's brother, sister-in-law, niece, and niece's husband lived another fifteen minutes away from the point of the accident.

The kind lady asked me if there was someone else to call, and I told her to call my son Joe. I heard her speak to him and inform him about the accident. After the calls, the lady handed me back my purse with my cell phone placed correctly in the side pocket. I could hear her calm and steady voice speak to me as I responded in a blank and nonfeeling state.

At this point, I had no emotions, no thought to ask for help. I was suspended in a state of nothingness. My husband and I were both pinned in the truck, helpless, and waiting for additional help to come to our rescue. I found out months later that the name of the kind lady who was the first to respond to our needs was Danielle, and her mother worked at the nearby Holiday Market.

## The Fire Departments and the Emergency Response Teams

Minutes seemed like hours, and I continued to wonder and worry about how much longer my husband could survive before more help came our way. I later found out that the Cool Fire Department, which was only two miles away, could not make the trip due to the heavy fog. The Georgetown Fire Department, which was ten miles away, was the first to respond, so it took about between twelve and fifteen minutes before I heard a male voice at my window.

I could see a tan jacket out of the side of my vision as I heard a male voice say with certainty, "Madame, my name is Ryan. I will be with you until more help comes." It was a Georgetown fireman, one of the first to show up to our rescue. I heard his voice, and it sounded like he was reporting to duty. I was so relieved because I knew he was in charge. When he told me his name was Ryan, I thought, *Oh, thank you, dear God, for sending me a sign.* My littlest grandson's name is Ryan, so I immediately saw it as a stroke of good fortune.

I asked about the other person, the one that hit us, if he was okay, even though I knew in my heart he had died in the moment of impact because I felt his spirit leave this earth. I heard someone answer me from a distance, as if he or she were on the opposite side of our truck. It was a woman's voice but not the same woman I had spoken to earlier. Her response was more firm and final when she said, "There is nothing we can do for him. He has gone. It is okay. He is in heaven now." Confused, I wondered if I heard her tell me that or if it was my own voice I was hearing.

Now I could hear additional fire trucks sounding their horns and the ambulance sirens in the distance. As the time passed, I wondered what was taking them so long to get there. After a while, I knew there were more firemen or rescue teams on the scene because I could hear conversations all around us. One rescue person was saying, "I think I'll try to get her out first." Then the Jaws of Life came crashing down directly above my head. One, two, three times I heard the slamming, powerful noise come crashing down before my passenger door was finally opened. I experienced no fear of the equipment hitting me; I sat very still. With the door opened, the rescue team very carefully removed me from our demolished truck. I remained motionless, and although my eyes were opened and I was conscious, I could not see anything around me. I could not see all the cars that were in the long traffic lines on both sides of the highway. I was placed on a gurney in a lying-down position. I remember asking someone if they could hand me my left hand so that I could hold on to it. It felt like my left arm was just dangling at my side and outside of the strap or belt they positioned me into for safety when on the gurney.

I knew that for Jean-Pierre the situation was far worse. He was trapped with the steering wheel locked up against his chest. His foot had gone through the floorboards and was deeply cut. The air bag had deployed, but the bottom part of it did not protect him. I remember that the firemen and rescue team did not drop a second once my door was opened; they immediately began to try to use the Jaws of Life on the driver's door. As they were lifting me onto the gurney, I could hear they were having a more difficult time trying to free my husband. It was taking them far longer than it had to release me. He continued to struggle for each breath and tried desperately to stay alive.

I heard someone say as they were lifting me into the ambulance, "Are you going to go ahead and take her?"

Someone else yelled back, "No, I think we will wait for him." I thought to myself, *Yes, that would be good,* because I wanted to be with my husband to be reassured he was still alive and breathing.

I did not recognize him as they lifted him into the ambulance and placed him next to me. He was wearing an oxygen mask, and they were beginning to start the IVs. But I knew in my heart it had to be him. There were four rescue persons in the back with us, or so it seemed. Everyone seemed to be rushing about, even with as little room as there was in the back of the ambulance. I tried to look over my shoulder to see if Jean-Pierre was okay, but the two rescue men were squatting down with their backs to me, and it looked like they were shielding me from seeing what was going on. I did not know it at the time, but I found out later form reading the fireman's report that they were administering advanced life support to my husband. Squatting down with their backs to me was their way of protecting me from seeing they were trying to save my husband's life.

The next thing I recall is the driver or someone in the front of the ambulance yelling back to us through a window, "We are almost there," meaning the trauma center at Sutter Hospital in Roseville, California. They pulled up to the emergency entrance of Sutter Trauma Center. I do not remember them taking me out of the ambulance.

My last thought in my memory bank of that night was looking down at my right leg and seeing someone's hands working large scissors and cutting off my brown corduroy pants. As the scissors began to reach the area around my knee, I realized I must have been in bad shape because no one had asked me to undress; they were doing it for me by cutting off my clothes. I must have blacked out or received medication because that is my last memory of that horrible night.

## My Husband's Perspective

On April 13, 2012, I interviewed my husband by asking some questions regarding the accident to capture his perspective.

**When you look back now on all that has happened to you with the accident, what do you know now that you did not know prior to the accident?**

"That's hard to say, but I'm more aware of other people now, the feelings of other people. Before, I did not care about people getting hurt; I just thought, *They will get better.* But now it hurts me, and I do not want to hear about other people getting hurt. I'm more sensitive to hearing about other people's injuries. I'm more conscious about it and more compassionate about it. Before, I would think, *Okay, big deal, he got hurt.* Now I can relate to their pain and suffering even though I cannot do anything about. It is just a good thing that there are doctors to help people with their pain and sufferings."

**What else is different now after the accident?**

"I'm looking more now at the end of my life. Before, I did not think about that; I just thought I would live, and live, and live, you know. Now I'm thinking I have five years or I have ten years. I'm looking more at what am I going to be like in five or ten years. I'm more aware of how I'm going to die or what's going to happen to me when it is the last years or something. I do not want to have a long disability where I cannot walk or stand up, and I fall down. That would be very terrible for me because I'm very active, and I do not want to let go of being active.

"It is kind of scary. I'm not afraid of dying because I died, and it was okay. It was just when I got out of the unconscious state,

I realized I was alive and was suffering with problems, and I was depending on people to give me a drink and to wash my face, and I was pooping ... and I could not do anything to turn me around, and I could not move my body anyway ... so I do not know what I was going to say. Oh, about dying, I would rather die quickly than have some long sickness."

**What has changed health-wise for you in your everyday living?**

"I'm living every day now. I did before, but now I'm not concerned about how much money I'm going to leave behind to others. I'm going to live life and enjoy every minute and spend as much as I can for me and you to have a good time to not suffer and whatever it takes to have a good life. I'm not going to be cold because I want to save money on gas, and I'm not going to be hungry because I want to save money. No, I'm just going to live, and that's how I feel like now, and that is what has changed for me. Before, I was worried about what is the cheapest way, and how can I fix things myself to save money. If I do something, it is because I want to do it and it is not going to affect my health, and if it is something I cannot do physically, I'm going to hire someone to do it."

**Has your strength changed?**

"Oh, yes, that has changed quite a bit because I have to take rests more often. I have to be sure to take my medication every day. Yes, physically, I have gone down quite a bit."

**How have you coped with the loss of your physical strength?**

"I want to go back and continue my exercises." (Since the writing of this, Jean-Pierre has returned to working out on the treadmill as a daily activity.) "When I exercise, I feel better about myself, and it just feels better all over. I did not have a lot of physical therapy activity after the accident. When I was healing from the surgeries, it was just strength-building exercises."

**How were you able to monitor your own pain medication once you returned home? Why did you make that decision, and how were you able to do that?**

"I have always monitored my own health, and I have always taken my own medicine regularly. I used my cell phone to wake me up each night to take my pain medication. I was journaling all of the times I took my medications, recording my blood pressure and blood oxygen levels multiple times a day. If I had any pain, I would also record this and any other symptoms I was experiencing. I had a hell of a time in the rehab center when one time the nurse forgot to give me my pain medication, so from then on, I began to record on my own and keep track for myself."

**How was your experience in the rehab center?**

"It was pretty good because slowly every day I was getting better. Slowly I did not need anyone to turn me around every day, and I could begin to do it on my own. I was able to sit up and things like that. The physical therapy was good because they were making me wash myself and go walk a little bit. In the beginning, it was pretty hard because I could not even stand up. As the weeks went on, I was doing much better doing things on my own. I do not recall how long I was in the rehab center though."

**Did it kind of overwhelm you when you came home and you had a whole hospital room in your living room area?**

"No, I took for granted that is what was needed at the time. I was positive things would gradually improve for us. I had a positive attitude in my mind that I was going to make it upstairs to my bedroom at some point in time. I was sure I was going to make it. I knew I was going to get out of Eskaton Rehab Center, and I knew that I would be getting out in good shape. I had made my mind up on that. I was not concerned that I did not have a car when I got home. I knew everything was going to be good again and that I would be back on my feet. I always had that in my mind. I never worried that I would be crippled or anything like that. I always knew in my mind it was going to be just like it was before the accident. At the rehab center, I knew things were going to be better because I had you there, and my daughter was with me also. I knew I was in good hands."

**What is the best advice you can give to someone who faces a sudden disability or injury?**

"You will get better, you are in good hands, and the doctors are doing everything they can to help you out. You are going to be better—maybe not as good as you were before, but you are going to be better. A positive attitude and a good spirit are what you need to get better. I always felt good once I realized what was going on and where I was because there were always people around me."

**What would you say was the most important thing in your recovery?**

"The most important thing to me in my recovery was my state of mind. In the rehab center, just knowing you were there with me—even with a broken arm, you were there with me. You got to have somebody there with you while you are recovering. To me, having people around me was very important for my well-being. You cannot be in an empty house with a nurse coming at a specific time every day to change your diapers. This is not good; you got to have people around you because that is very important."

**Were you surprised by how many people were there to help you?**

"No, I was not surprised because I always knew my family would be there. I was hoping they would be there, and they were. It is very important to have your family around you and help you."

**Was there a point right after the accident that was a pivotal point for you?**

"Just after the accident, I could not breathe. I was hoping they would take me out of that wreck because I was pinned down and I could not breathe, and I kept telling the fireman, 'I cannot breathe,' and I couldn't. I tried to take a breath, and I couldn't. I lost consciousness quite a few times. The first time was right after the hit; I was out. Then when I was out of the unconscious state there was nobody around, and you were sitting there, and I said, 'Are you okay?' and you said, 'I'm hurt.' I do not remember exactly what you said, but you were talking, so that meant you were okay, and you were right there with me, and then I passed out again. The next thing I remember, I tried to breathe, and I could not breathe, and they were cutting the metal on the truck off. I passed out again, and I remember I was in the ambulance, and the guy said, 'We are going to do everything we can.' ... Honey, I do not want to talk about it anymore."

At this point, the interview ended because it was too upsetting to go on with the interview.

## A Loss of Time

I do not remember if it was the next day or later that evening when I realized I was in a hospital bed in the ICU and my entire left arm from the shoulder down to my fingertips was heavily bandaged. A nurse was saying to whoever was in my room, "She better not move her arm like that." I knew there were people in the room because I could hear them walking about. I thought they might be relatives of our family but was uncertain. Even though my eyes were opened, I could not see clearly enough to identify anyone, and I did not think anyone was addressing me directly.

I could hear my son Joe on the cell phone a short distance away from my bed with his back turned away from me. He was talking to someone and saying, "They do not think Jean-Pierre is going to make it." Joe was upset; I could hear it in his voice as he spoke. He was breaking down, and his voice began to crack. Weeks later, I was informed that my whole family was there to support us—my brothers, my sons, family friends, and my husband's family.

Very soon after the accident and while in the hospital trauma center, I vaguely recall a police officer at my bedside trying to ask me questions. He had blond hair, and his metal badge was shining from the bed light against his dark blue uniform. He asked several questions, but the one question I remember is him asking me if I wore a seatbelt. I was either so drugged up or in a state of shock and feeling completely numb that I immediately raised my hospital gown to show him my seatbelt's imprint in dark blue and purple bruises that crossed over my body from my shoulder to my waist, exposing both breasts. He nodded, and that's all I remember of his presence. I think he left immediately after my little demonstration. I think in my mind at that moment, no one was going to make me wrong for the accident that killed one man and left my husband fighting for his life.

## Injuries and Sudden Disabilities

It was not until the next day, when my husband's doctor came into the room to speak to me, that I fully realized what was going on to some degree. He was a large, heavyset man with graying hair. He said, "Mrs. Korn, I went in to see your husband, and he is in the state of dying. We took him to surgery and removed three liters of blood from his heart lining." The surgeon continued to speak and provide details for me, but I became nauseated and began to vomit into a basin someone had placed near my mouth. He continued with, "We had to bring him back to the operating room because he continues to hemorrhage. We did not know where that was coming from. We discovered additional bleeding in his large ribs. A few hours after the second surgery, he began to swell, so we had to open him up to prevent additional swelling." I did not know at the time the meaning of "open him up" meant making an incision from his neck to his groin and leaving him open in this state for five days. In medical terms, this incision is called a "zipper" cut.

I continued to dry heave every time the doctor further explained my husband's health status. I could not take any more details because it was all just too much to absorb. In just a matter of hours, our whole life had changed and was upside down. I managed to interrupt the doctor as he continued to tell me the gory details of my husband's health status. I said, "I cannot hear anything more. Can you just tell me if he is going to live, and will he improve?"

His response was short and quick. "I cannot tell you that

right now." He left the room as fast as he had arrived. Suddenly my nausea subsided, but I was being given a morphine drip, and I believe that may have also contributed to my being physically and emotionally sick.

It was weeks later that I finally realized my husband had sustained two major surgeries within hours and had been left open from the chest to the pelvis for approximately five days due to body swelling. His injuries included a crushed chest with a contusion to the heart and hemorrhaging in the space of the chest between where the heart is located and the lungs are. He sustained massive blood loss from his internal injuries. In addition, he had a severe cut on his leg where his foot went through the floorboard.

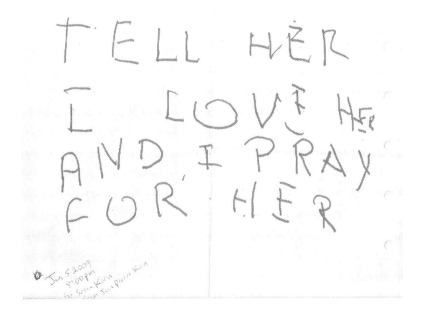

This letter from my husband was written three days after the accident. I never received this letter, maybe due to all the confusion going on during his immediate recovery period of trying to save his life. I found it months later while putting away all our paperwork accumulated from staying at three facilities. I do wish I could have seen it when he wrote it so that I would have known he was well enough to write it and wanted to send it to me. I think it demonstrates the profound weakness he was experiencing, as well as the courage he had to state what was on his mind during this crisis.

## My Immediate Thoughts: Trying to Remain Sane

While in the ICU at the trauma center, I began to hallucinate, and as more people and family members began to fill my room, I became confused. I could not make out anyone's facial features. I thought I saw my younger son, Zachary, standing a distance behind me, and I thought he had his fingers in his mouth and was biting his nails. I thought my two brothers, Anthony and Michael, were in the room, but I was not sure. The only person I was sure of was my son Joe.

My mind began to play tricks on me as I began to hallucinate, thinking I was at a Christmas party and that my visitors were tiny elves in the room with green-and-red outfits and white fur trimming on their sleeves and hem lines. They were moving all about, as with excitement. I happened to say to my son Joe, "I'm confused. I do not know what is going on. What is happening?"

It was immediately after that statement that I heard Joe make an announcement. "All right now, everyone out of the room." I did not know who he was directing his statement to. As the days passed, Joe informed me that I was asking for people who had been dead for twenty years. To this day, I do not know who I was asking to see.

Every now and then, I would recall what the doctor said to me about my husband's health status. I began to pray continually, night and day, every waking moment, for his well-being. I prayed like I had never prayed before. When I would discover that I had dozed off for a while and then awakened, I would continue my praying. I wanted him to live more than anything. I did not care about my own health or safety. I was only fixed on his recovery and having him be strong enough to get through this critical time. I do not recall eating anything in the ICU or having a tray of food placed in front of me. I do not recall any nurse or doctor informing me I was scheduled for surgery on my left arm three days later.

I have no recall of ever signing a consent form. Could it be that my son Joe signed for me and gave permission for my surgery? I do not know to this day how that all came about. I have no recall of being prepped for surgery, going to surgery, or being in the recovery room. For three days, my life seemed like a haze, and I was suspended into nothingness. I was not aware of night or day or what time or hour it was, and nothing seemed to matter. The only thing I could hold on to was to ask God to answer my prayers and save my husband's life.

## What I Do Remember

Apparently, the hospital waited three days so that a hand surgeon could perform my surgery. I do remember a doctor telling me his name when I was in the operating room. I could not pronounce it correctly, and he tried repeating it to me three times so that I would get it right. Looking back, it was a good decision to wait for a hand surgeon because of the severity of my left arm and wrist having multiple breaks. It was not until much later that I discovered that after the operation I had seven pins in my left hand to my lower forearm, and a titanium rod placed in my upper arm with three screws. Two screws were placed under the clavicle, and one screw was placed lower down on my upper arm to hold the rod in place. My fingers were so bruised they looked like little Vienna sausages. My saving grace for the immediate time frame was not suffering with any pain since I was still on heavy drugs.

## Pain Medication

The good thing about medication is it can take away the immediate pain wherever you hurt, and everywhere else in your body for that matter. When I was finally placed in my hospital bed, one of the first things I can recall is the nurse saying to me, "Here is a morphine drip button. When you hurt, all you have to do is press this button, and the morphine will go into your body." Thank God there is a limit to how much you can administer to yourself because I pressed that button until I was asleep. I did so for the first few days of the injury and then after the operation.

I was in terrible pain and emotionally and mentally could not tolerate any pain on top of this horrible ordeal. When it was time to be off the IV of morphine, I was given morphine pills to ease the pain in my arm and fingers. The swelling in my left hand, arm, and fingers was tremendous, like a rubber glove blown up, and my fingers were completely black and blue with bruises. The swelling was so bad in my fingers you could hardly recognize them. I had come close to losing my left arm from the accident. It was months later that I was informed that my left arm, wrist, and hand had gone through the dashboard of our truck, crushing many bones. The upper arm had an open fracture close to the shoulder area.

Weeks later, I tried to reduce the amount of pain medication once I saw my husband at the rehab center because I wanted to be more aware of his well-being and health status. I remember withdrawing from the hard drugs and fighting the withdrawals. I was soaking wet from perspiration, and you could literally ring me out like a wash rag, but I was determined to get off the hard stuff. The withdrawals lasted several days, and then I began to feel a little better but very tired from what my body had gone through. It was very hard to endure the pain in my arm, but I wanted to be alert to see my husband and to be a support system to him once he arrived at the rehab center with me.

# PART II:

# THE RECOVERY PERIOD AND REHABILITATION

### Leaving My Husband Behind Fighting for His Life

By Wednesday, six days later, I was considered stable and ready to be transferred to Kaiser Hospital in Roseville, California. Before my transfer, I was asked by a nurse if I wanted to see my husband before being transferred. Yes, of course I wanted to see him; it had been too many days without knowing how he was. I considered this good news because if he had died, someone would have informed me. However, I was not prepared for or prewarned about what I was about to see. First, I was surprised to realize we were only a few rooms down from each other. *How come no one informed me of this?* I thought. *How come I did not know enough to ask where he was?* The drugs had done what they were supposed to do. They were keeping me without pain and without feelings or a sense of others' well-being. I was in my own dream world trying to get through each day, even if they all seemed to flow together without meaning.

When the nurse wheeled me into his room, I could not believe my eyes and thought my brain was playing tricks on me. I was sure the pain medication was messing with my mind. I could not believe what I was seeing.

My husband was in an upright position with his bed rolled into a sitting position. His hands were tied to the bed rails. He was in excruciating pain, and his breathing was labored. He looked like Jesus nailed to the cross and in deep agony. I could hardly stand to look at him, and yet my heart was breaking. I knew this might be my last time to see him alive.

I asked him if he wanted to pray, and he said yes by nodding his head. I said the Our Father and the Hail Mary out loud in a soft and steady voice. I was trying desperately to hold up and be strong as I was thinking to myself, *Oh, dear God, please tell me this is a nightmare and I will soon wake up*. Again reality set in, and I could not tolerate seeing him in so much pain and distress. He was unable to pray out loud with me.

I did not or could not kiss him good-bye because I could not tolerate seeing him like that. It was the vision of a nightmare before my eyes, only I knew I was not dreaming. This was for real, and it was my husband in torture before my eyes. I was numb on heavy drugs as I realized he was still struggling to stay alive even after so many days had passed. I was going to be transferred to a rehab center, and I wondered if my husband was ever going to improve and survive this terrible ordeal. He did not know it, but I left my heart with him that day as I continued to pray for his recovery.

## Transferring to Kaiser Permanente Roseville Medical Center

Many strange things happened during the time Jean-Pierre and I were separated from each other. We each had our own battles to overcome. I was always about two weeks ahead of him in recovery and being released from the hospitals. All in all, we both journeyed through three medical facilities: Sutter Trauma Center, Kaiser Roseville Hospital, and Eskaton Rehabilitation, a skilled nursing facility.

I stayed in Kaiser Roseville for a few days before being transferred again. I was not hearing from my husband's doctors about his health status. I knew his daughters would make sure he got the treatment and care he needed. They were able to communicate with the nursing staff around the clock.

My son Joseph came to visit me every day and brought a beautiful bouquet of flowers for me. The physical therapists wasted no time in coming to visit with me. One of my first exercises was to try to move my fingers. She said it was very important that I continue to move my fingers, even for just a little bit every hour. She was also helpful in trying to help me get out of bed and walk a few steps. I was carrying the IV pole with me when she said, "Your son is just outside of your room door. Why don't we surprise him and show him you are walking a bit?" I agreed, and as we went through the door, I smiled at my son and walked very slowly past him. I could tell he was quite moved at seeing me trying to walk again. It had been days since the accident, and I was now up and trying to move a bit.

## Oh No—Not Diapers!

It had been days, and in none of that time did I feel like going to the bathroom. In fact, I have no recall of that feeling until one evening I was getting the notion of having to move my bowels, and it came on quickly and instantly. I called for the nurse with my bed light. It seemed like an eternity before a young lady came in to see what I wanted. I believe she was an aide, and she became very flustered when I asked to go to the bathroom. She said, "Oh, my goodness, you are going to need a bedpan." (Yes, that would be right—and right now, please!) She then said she would need a face mask and gloves for her hands as she hurriedly looked in the cabinets and then abruptly left the room after placing a bedpan under me. Well, I had not gone in days, and believe me, it was explosive! I could tell the pan was filling up rapidly and beginning to overflow, or so I thought from my position lying down on my back. I thought, *Oh, holy God, please help me! (And where is that nurse?)*

I rang for the nurse again, and almost immediately, a male RN came in. I felt sheer horror as I looked at him in disbelief. *Can this get any worse?* I thought. *I have to tell him what happened, and he may very well be the one to clean me up.* I just wanted to die at that very moment. I gave him such a look that he said, "What? What is wrong? What is it?" I said, "I've messed my bed," in a voice filled with shame and terror. Being a professional of high standing, he said, "Is that all?" He quickly put on gloves, moved over to my side of the bed, and quickly removed that bedpan and the soiled sheets. He cleaned me up in no time with the swiftness of a true professional. In the meantime, the aide came back into the room with her hands waving in the air wearing rubber gloves, and now she was wearing a face mask. I was pleased she located them, but it came at a high price as I was sitting my in own mess before the nurse came in.

The male RN and the aide exchanged some words, and before I knew it, the aide was trying to put a diaper on me. It did not fit, and she yelled out to the male RN as he was leaving my room, "Bring the big blue ones," meaning big blue diapers because these ones did not fit. As I lay on my back looking up at the bright lights over my head, I thought to myself, *Oh, dear God, what has happened to my life?* Here when I did not think life could get any worse, I was now being placed in adult diapers—and the big ones at that.

As the little aide struggled to put the blue diapers on me, I looked up at the light in the ceiling of my room and thought it was as if time had moved forward twenty years, and now I was in diapers like an elderly person. I kept wondering what had happened to my life. Another interesting thing happened to me. I began to think my son Zachary would be calling me, and I would tell him what had happened. Just as the aide left my room, my phone rang, and sure enough it was Zachary calling me to see how I was. I started to cry and said, "I just messed my bed. And now they put me in a diaper."

He began to chuckle and said, "That's okay, Mom. I understand because you are a proud woman, and I know how difficult that is for you, but it is only temporary." I was so relieved he had called me so that I could share my dilemma with someone who I would be able to talk to at that very moment. I did feel better after he reassured me it was only for temporary reasons.

The next day when my therapist came into the room, I told her about my experience because there was no way to hide the big blue diapers I was wearing. She informed me this was a common problem with most people because after a trauma of such magnitude, having surgery, and taking medications, it takes the body a few days to settle down and relieve itself. It would have been nice to have been forewarned about that so that I would have known what I was in for. I'll never forget the kindness and professional manner the male RN gave to me to make feel like a person again and a lady. He so swiftly gave me back my dignity. He said to me that horrible night, "Sometimes God makes us lie down so that we can look up." I later discovered he was a physician in the Philippines and an RN here in this country. He also told me he carried rosary beads with him at all times. He lifted them out of his pocket to show me his devotion to his religion. I will never forget that awful event that took place and the wonderful nurse who gave me back my dignity.

## A Daughter's Love and Commitment

When Jean-Pierre's daughters, Michelle and Karla, received word of our accidents, they immediately made arrangements to fly out from South Carolina to be by our side. His other daughter who lived in Santa Rosa was immediately at our bedside once she received the news.

Once they arrived, I knew Jean-Pierre's daughters were by his side night and day holding a vigil over his bedside. I was happy and relieved they were there because due to my own injuries, I could not be there. I knew they would try everything in their power to keep their father alive and to keep up his spirits.

Apparently, Jean-Pierre did not like his food and had no appetite, so when it was time for him to have solid foods, his daughter went out and bought all kinds of gourmet food for him to feast on. She bought him wonderful creamy, rich cheeses, French breads, olives, and duck-liver pâté, which he loved. Anything one could imagine, he had it in front of him. I think she purchased about three hundred dollars of this highly priced gourmet food.

His daughters slept in his room and were available for any instructions or details that were given by the healthcare professionals who were tending to their father's care. After ten days of night-and-day care, Michelle had to go back home to tend to her family and their catering business. Karla continued to stay with her father. She was determined not to leave his side until he was on his feet again. She cared for him night and day and kept a journal of his recovery.

## A Son's Devotion

My saving grace was my son Joe who called each day to see how I was prior to coming over to visit me after his work each day. He would bring me a lunch or dinner from the nearby restaurants. He had informed me there was a delicious kosher deli nearby where they had wonderful food and especially wonderful homemade chicken noodle soup. Did I want some? Oh, boy, did I want some. The food at the rehab center was not terrible; they managed to serve at least one decent meal a day. Breakfast always had some form of hot cereal like oatmeal or cream of wheat, a cup of tea or coffee, toast, and then a strip of bacon or egg. Lunch or dinner was usually okay to eat, but if I had my druthers, I would rather have something from the nearby restaurants; it was just tastier. I knew chicken noodle soup was what the doctor ordered for nutrition and strength. I relished its favor, and it satisfied my taste buds. One day, I would have a corn beef sandwich with kosher dill pickle, or an order of fried shrimp, or possibly a Cobb salad. To me, nothing looked finer than seeing my son come through the doors of that rehab center with a white bag in hand. I would meet him in the grand lobby with my wheelchair, and we would eat together at one of the large dining tables. If it was not for my son, I may not have had something to look forward to each day.

## The Value of Friends

Many friends and family members came to our bedsides to wish us well and offer hope for a speedy recovery. Once I was transferred to the rehab center and my health status was more stable, more friends came from our Gold Hound Association and their women's auxiliary association, The Red Hats Ladies. Many of our friends and family members brought flowers and a good ear for listening to me. I sure hope I was making sense at that time. Visiting with family and friends is a delight when you are hospital bound and cannot go out and about on your own or leave the hospital or rehab facility. You are stuck there whether you like it or not, and the days can seem mighty long without visitors. I really enjoyed the long talks and visit of our friends who came by to see me and ask about Jean-Pierre.

I remember at one point my son Zachary said to me on the phone, "I love you, and I'm glad you are still alive." Although my family made efforts to visit often, my son Zachary and his children lived three hours away. However, they did come and visit a few times. As my son wheeled me out into the fresh warm air of the front garden of the rehab center, I had joy in knowing I could see my grandsons for a short visit and share a few pleasant times together. It was important to me to keep a good, positive attitude around my grandchildren, children, and friends. I did not want them to feel sorry for me or to think for one moment that I might be staying there for good. No way. I was getting out as soon as I was able to do things to some degree on my own. But first I had to get out of the wheelchair and move on to a walking cane, so I needed to regain my strength.

One fine morning, my friend Wanda called me at the rehab center and let me know she was coming to visit. She asked what I would like for her to bring me to eat. Oh boy, here was my chance for something special. I immediately responded, "A hamburger, fries, and a strawberry milkshake." What else could be on my mind but good old-fashioned American fast food? As the noon hour approached, she arrived with the wonderful little bag she was carrying just for me! We ate lunch together and sat in the grand lobby, and I cannot tell you how wonderful and tasty that meal was. You know, your body craves anything that will bring you back to your old self, and a hamburger, French fries, and strawberry milkshake were just what the doctor ordered. Besides bringing me a much-needed lunch, Wanda brought me some little gifts, one being a pink bunny rabbit. It so reminded me of the blue bunny rabbit I had at home. Interesting enough, I had been thinking about the blue little rabbit sitting in my bedroom at home, and I had begun to miss it. When I'm hurting, it is comforting to me to snuggle up to something warm, soft, and cozy. Wanda's pink little bunny did the trick for me, and I remember being very happy about receiving it.

Another time when I was traveling to visit Jean-Pierre and staying at my son's home in Sacramento, I needed a ride home since I could not drive with my injuries. Wanda had said she would come to pick me up when I was ready. I had asked her because it was a Friday, generally her day off, and she lived not too far from the rehab center. Well, it was particularly bad weather, and the rain was pouring down something awful. The clock in my husband's hospital room showed it was several hours past five o'clock in the evening. I was becoming worried about Wanda driving in the horrible weather, and then she arrived all in a rush and out of breath. She had worked that particular Friday and was fighting the bad weather and traffic all the way. I was very grateful that she came to my rescue to drive me back to my son's home. This was the sign of a loyal and true friend.

Another time, Linda, my childhood friend who lived in Oregon, was visiting the Bay Area and wanted to see for herself that I was okay. She offered to take me to order new eyeglasses since mine had been broken in the accident. I had been going around without any glasses for three weeks, so her offer to help me was great. I could not make up my mind about which glasses looked appropriate. I was still on pain medication, and my mind did not seem clear at the time. Linda was very helpful in selecting a pair of glasses that looked appropriate for my age and right for the shape of my face. Again, a dear friend came to my rescue.

After a month of being at home, four of our close friends came by to visit us. We were still very much in the recovery period and welcomed seeing our friends. What we did not realize was they had planned to bring enough food prepared by them to help sustain us for one week. There was food for us all to share during their visit, but they had also prepared a lot of food that needed only to be placed in the freezer until a later time. I was so humbled by their thoughtfulness and kindness. Our friends and family members were wonderful to us during this difficult time. They were truly angels on earth for all their kindness and generosity.

*Optimism is the faith that leads to achievement.*
*Nothing can be done without hope and confidence.*
—Helen Keller

## Eskaton Senior Residences and Services: Off to Rehab

A few days later, the hospital personnel were making arrangements for me to be transferred to a rehabilitation center for further physical therapy and recovery. By now, I had been assigned a Kaiser orthopedic doctor and he was the chief of the Orthopedics Department at Kaiser Roseville. The first day I met him, he was very nice to me and told me that the other doctor had done a good job on my arm and hand at Sutter. He told me I would be transferred to a rehabilitation center for further treatment and to continue my physical therapy exercises. I did not know it at the time, but he was a very talented and gifted doctor and has done wonders helping his patients improve through his surgical techniques. I heard many compliments about him from his other patients when in the waiting room. They spoke so highly of him and his excellent work as a surgeon. One patient said he was a saint. I knew in my heart I had to trust someone, so I put all my trust and respect in my doctor. He did not fail me.

I learned from my doctor that my arm and hand had so many breaks they could not put some of the smaller bones together. They had counted nine breaks in my lower arm and hand and one break in my upper arm, which broke completely through.

There were only twelve rehab centers, and out of the top

three, he was going to send me to the number-one facility. He said they were number one due to the level of physical therapy care they provided. He said, "They never do anything without contacting me first for approval. I like that." Just as he was talking to me, he turned into a great big chocolate Hershey bar. You know, the kind that has brown wrapping with the foil. I think those are the ones that have almonds in them. I decided I better tell someone what I was experiencing, so I told the doctor. His response was interesting, as he stated, "Well, that's kind of scary because I eat a lot of chocolate!" I knew if he was not concerned, then I didn't need to be. He is the only person who ever turned into a chocolate bar on me!

I remember one of my girlfriends and her daughter came to visit with me just before my transfer from Kaiser to the rehab center. They had brought me my Christmas presents and some medical supplies one needs when staying in a hospital environment. I was thrilled to get a pale blue bathrobe and slippers to match. It brought me back to that old feeling of receiving a new robe and slippers whenever being hospitalized. They were both happy to see me and tried to be cheery, but my waking thoughts were still consumed with worrying about Jean-Pierre and his health status.

Days were passing, and I did not get any word about his status. I was becoming agitated, and I do not know if it was the drugs taking effect or not, but my girlfriend and her daughter were telling me they would be following me over to the rehab center that I was now being transferred to. I was starting to feel uncertain about being transferred to a place I was unfamiliar with and concerned about how long I would be there and what it would be like. I had heard so many stories about skilled nursing facilities that the idea of going there started to consume my thoughts.

Unfortunately, my behavior was misread by my girlfriend, and it was months later that I found out she was feeling dismissed by me. No, it was more like I was concerned about my transfer and feeling lots of anxiety and agitation. Under the influence of heavy drugs, I found that I had little patience to deal with a lot of chatter and fast movements. I do not know if it was because I had so much on my mind like my husband dying or it was the pain medications. In any event, I was beginning to feel exhausted and wanted to be just left alone with my thoughts.

My son had made financial arrangements for me to be transferred by ambulance to Eskaton Rehabilitation Center. It was a skilled nursing facility as well, and I had wild thoughts about what to expect. I knew from previous experience with my mother and other relatives that the nursing-home food was awful, to say the least. I was just hoping the nursing care would be appropriate and acceptable. Both my parents in their final stages of life had been in skilled nursing facilities, and although they were adequate, there was still much left to be desired.

Before I knew it, the transportation ambulance arrived and my thoughts of "what's next" started to stir within me. One of my main concerns was how long I was going to be in the rehab center. What was that decision based on? And most important, was I going to like it there or wish I were dead instead?

My girlfriend and her daughter drove behind the ambulance to follow me there. They were trying to be cheery and helpful, but all the changes that had taken place in the past several days were just becoming too much for me to bear. I was now even further away from Jean-Pierre because he was still at the Sutter Trauma Center in the ICU. I still had not heard from his doctors but was receiving here and there small bits of information from family members who either called on the phone or came to visit me.

Once I arrived at the rehab center, I was placed in a two-bed hospital room. My bed was further from the entrance door. An elderly lady was in the bed next to me, and she was very quiet, kept to herself, and did not speak or ask me any questions. At bedtime, the confused patients with dementia would scream in the middle of the night, "Someone help me!" They would scream this nonstop until a nurse's aide would come in to comfort them. Another patient would pound on his bed table with his fists into the early morning hours. These behaviors caused sleep interruptions for me, and it went on for days. I started to wonder why someone wasn't giving these troubled patients some medication to have them sleep at night. After several days, my wish came true, and it finally settled down at night so that I could get some much-needed rest.

In a couple of days, they moved me another room right next to the one I was originally placed in. My new roommate was a younger woman than the one before and more talkative. She wasted no time in informing me that the woman who was in the bed before me had died in it a few days ago. *Oh that's great*, I thought to myself. My new bed was near a long, narrow window, and I could tell it had been raining for days. I was somewhat pleased I was warm and inside but wondered what the rest of the world was doing. It was cold and damp outside for most of the month of January that year. I could hear the rain beating against the window and was glad for the comfort of my bed. Even at this time, life seemed to have no purpose for me.

## Night Shift in Rehab

I had been troubled about the other person who was involved in the accident with us. I did not know him, but my husband had spoken to him once or twice before the accident ever occurred. Living in a small community like Cool, one comes across almost everyone now and again. It appeared that this person owned an auto repair business here in our town, and my husband had brought one of our cars to him for repairing. The other unusual thing was this person was living with his girlfriend on a piece of property that was right next to ours. Our properties are each five acres with fence lines separating our parcels. I did not know this at the time of the accident and had never met this man before. I was very troubled to know that someone had lost his life and that I had witnessed his last moment on earth. Although family and friends tried to comfort me by saying, "It was not your fault," it did little to help.

The man who died was well known in town, and at least five people informed me that he frequented the local saloon. The CHP report that we received months later stated he was under the influence of alcohol when the accident occurred. I do not know if he fell asleep at the wheel or he could not see due to the fog or if alcohol played a role in his decision making; I only know he is no longer with us.

So while I was in the rehab center, the man who died at the scene of the accident was really starting to bother me. I felt like he and I had some unresolved issues to settle between us. One of the nights I could not sleep, I went to the grand lobby and went on the computer there to search for this person. His photo came up on the obituary news, and this was the first time I was able to see what he looked like. He was a big man with a big smile on his face, and he was dressed in Western wear with a large, light-colored cowboy hat. He was standing near a fence in the country, and a horse was in the near background. As I saw his face, I had a talk with him. I told him how sorry I was that he had died, and how I wish I could have changed what happened. It helped to put a face to a name, but I still felt terrible about his death. I wondered to myself that night if I would ever find peace with what happened.

I found myself having difficulty sleeping at night. It appeared unless you were with the physical therapy department doing exercises and building up your strength, there was little to do but sleep or sit quietly and watch all the activity going on outside your room. In the beginning when my nights and days were mixed up, I had a sweet night-shift nurse's aide who would keep me company. We talked about her career and working for a healthcare facility and all the things one chats about when one is lonely and seeking companionship. I enjoyed our little talks until I feel asleep.

When I was able to get out of bed, I discovered I would wake up at about 3:00 a.m. each night. I got the notion one day to wheel myself into the grand lobby and use their computer. When the nurse saw me, she said, "Mrs. Korn, what are you doing?" I said, "I cannot sleep, and I'm doing to use the computer." After that first time, I was known for going to the lobby in the middle of the night to write e-mails to my friends and to just have something to do to overcome the boredom. After an hour or so, I would wheel myself back to my room and fall asleep again until morning.

## Bath Time

One of things I liked least about my stay at the rehab center was I had to take a shower. I enjoy bathtubs so much more. I was wheeled to the shower room, which was in another section of the building on the second floor. The one shower in our sleep area was under construction, so we could only use the one upstairs. I sat in a shower chair as the aide helped me get undressed, and then she would wheel me into the shower. There was a cold draft, and when the water was not on a particular part of my body, I would feel a chill. The whole ordeal was unpleasant for me due to the cold draft. Then I was wheeled the long distance back to my room with wet hair.

Having a shower at the rehab center was a necessary evil, and I really do not know that it could have been made any better or more pleasant since I could not use my arm. I had little mobility to wash myself and my hair. The worst part during the shower was sitting in the plastic chair that had a large hole in it similar to a toilet seat. Yes, the aide would use the shower hose to spray right up into the hole of the chair, and I was washed by the power of the water spray in the genitals area. Believe me, this was no fun and one of the main reasons I wanted to get my life back so that I could manage to clean myself in the way I was used to … not some hose on full blast up the yazoo.

All in all, I was very surprised how much skilled nursing facilities had changed for the better since my mother was in one twenty years before. It was in the 1980s when my mother was in and out of nursing homes due to breast cancer. She was receiving chemotherapy treatments and lived too far away to go to the doctor appointments on her own. She stayed at two skilled nursing facilities in Santa Rosa, California, and they were both pretty close to my place of work. The facilities always seemed so cold, and the staff seemed to always be in a hurry. They were sometimes unfriendly and stayed pretty much to themselves. Most nursing facilities in those days had an odor of urine and death, and I dreaded visiting.

However, when I was transferred to Eskaton, it was a very different place. The nurses all seemed friendly and willing to help in any way possible. They tried to cheer me up and many times had a smile on their face. The one thing I liked very much was their ability to get to know me as a person, always willing to hear what I had to say and to do whatever necessary to make my stay comfortable. I did not detect any odor while staying there either.

## Rehab Food Service

After a week, I received a visit from the dietitian. His concern was that all my trays were being returned untouched except for the breakfast trays. I tried to be as polite as possible when I let him know I do not eat like this. He asked me what I would like to eat. I mentioned a piece of fresh fruit like a banana, or strawberries, or a handful of nuts like almonds, and raw carrots. Any food items that were fresh would be nice. I said I realized the food is prepared for the elderly who many times have to have pureed meals because they cannot always chew and bite, but that was not what I needed. After my visit with the dietitian, I noticed the kitchen made an effort to bring more fresh fruits and raw vegetables, but there was still so much room for improvement on the food trays they served.

## Surgical Wound Care

I believe you are still in charge when it comes to who cleans your wounds and how it is done—meaning, in a gentle and kind manner. The only time I experienced some difficulty in communicating was when a visiting nurse came in to change and clean the dressings on my arm. I was naturally guarded of my injured arm and fearful of experiencing any more pain than needed. The surgical dressing nurse was not available, and the visiting nurse was going to clean my wound and change my bandages. I mentioned to her that it was a painful experience. I said, "If it hurts too much, would you stop?" She acted like she never heard me and continued to clean my wound with the same amount pressure.

It began to hurt something awful, and she still continued to clean my wound after I mentioned it was painful. It got to the point where I told her to stop, that I would wait for the other nurse to come and clean my wounds. She did stop at that point, and I could tell she was upset with me for refusing her care. I felt I had a right to request who I wanted to care for my wounds and dress them. I did not care at that moment about her feelings, particularly since she never acknowledged my feelings of how painful the procedure was for me.

After a few hours, the surgical nurse came in to clean and dress my arm. She was excellent and never hurt me at all with the cleaning procedure. I thanked her and asked why the other person did not respond to me. Her response surprised me when she said, "Well, most of the people here are senile and do not know what is going on, so she probably was just ignoring you." I never again allowed the visiting nurse to clean my wound.

## Waiting to See the Doctor

I had a work history of working for Kaiser Permanente for many years, so when I heard there was a KP doctor who came to visit patients there, I was thrilled. I could not wait to meet him and make a connection with my old employer. He was a quiet man and listened to my concerns about medications and the inability to sleep at night. KP also had a visiting nurse who came to visit their patients to see how their care was going. When I met this nurse, I could not help but to put my arms around her and hug her. Just knowing there was someone there who cared about us from Kaiser Permanente made me feel not alone.

## Physical Therapy at Rehab

Again, I cannot say enough about the men and women who dedicate their lives to helping others. However, they cannot make miracles happen; they can only lead the way to help us improve and get past all the pain to gain the strength of our body parts to get back to normal or as close to normal as possible. They devote the time and effort to show us the way and how to work out with the different equipment to regain our strength and mobility. When they say "Do this three times a day," then that is what it takes to improve. If your body freezes or refuses to move, it is not their fault because it is our responsibility to do whatever is possible to improve. I used to say I wanted to be a spry old woman with all parts workings. Well, guess what? Life got in the way, and now I have to really work at it if I want all my body parts to work and move in the right direction and be there when I need them. I have learned that how you treat your body determines how well it will treat you years later. It is a hard lesson to learn after the wear and the tear of hard work and going beyond what your body can handle comfortably.

Physical therapy plays a role in most surgeries, and I have always paid very close attention to following all instructions and exercises. I believe most of my good results have come directly from following the doctors' and physical therapists' instructions. You have to get through the pain and not give up in order to gain the best possible results.

Yes, it is painful and exhausting, but as you master each step of the recovery period in physical therapy, there is a big gain at the end. It is like taking a course in karate; at each step, you receive a different color belt as you progress and succeed. Well, in this case, it maybe a different color squeeze sponge, a different color plastic stretch strap, or more weights to lift, but each new step tells you your strength, body, and muscle tone are improving, and I'm all for that.

The physical therapist came to see me on the second day of my arrival at the rehab center. She was very nice and asked me how I felt. Each day, they would come into my room and have me do exercises with my fingers and hands if I could, and they would assist me in walking a few steps. After three days, I was getting discouraged; it seemed like such a slow process. However, my PT informed me that on the first day, I needed help getting out of bed, and I walked only eleven feet. On my third day, I no longer needed help getting out of bed, and I walked thirty feet, which in her opinion was very good. Yes, I guess it was, but it seemed like such a long road ahead for me. I wondered if I would ever get back to my normal self again.

I was labeled a "fall risk" because I had a history of falling and losing my balance. This is a title that gets you some recognition whether you want it or not. In the rehab center, my means of transportation was either a wheelchair or a Hemi Walker, which I really liked. It is like half a walker, and you place it on your good side and use it like a cane to help you walk and keep your balance. There was no way I could go fast, but then fast was not in my vocabulary anymore. As one PT said, "Fast does not always mean better."

My first day being taken to the physical therapy department, the physical therapist threw me a curve ball when she said, "Mrs. Korn, what if I was to say to you your arm will never get any better than what it is now? What would you say to me?" It did not take me long to respond. I was curious as to why she had said this statement to me when it was my first day in the PT department. I replied, "Well, I guess it is still my arm, and it is still attached." We worked together starting from that point.

Along with singing with the other patients and playing games like bean bag "tit, tat, toe," in which I got a perfect score, a first time ever for the PT department, we worked hard at regaining my balance and strength in my overall body. My arm was nowhere near doing any work with it. I was just learning to walk again on those balance bars to prevent myself from falling. While at the rehab center in PT, they showed me how to walk up and down stairs again by using balance bars. They showed me how to prepare a meal in their make-believe kitchen using only one arm. For example, instead of lifting a heavy pan filled with water and moving it from the sink to the counter, fill a pitcher, place the empty pot on the stove top, and then fill it. They showed me how to rearrange my kitchen by moving the microwave to the countertop or sliding the filled casserole dish closer to the microwave before placing it in there. There were many ways PT helped me to understand new ways to do something instead of the traditional way I had been so used to in the past. These approaches helped me to regain a sense of independence again.

## God Visits Nursing Homes Too

I had been in the rehab center for a couple of days when one morning about six a.m. I was awakened by a man of the cloth. He was an elderly man in his eighties, and I woke up and saw his dark gown and the collar he was wearing. I immediately thought he was a priest and said to him in a desperate voice, "Oh, Father, I'm so glad you are here." He corrected me in a kind and gentle manner and said, "Oh, I'm not a priest. I'm a pastor." I said, "But you are a Christian, and you believe in God?" He said, "Yes."

I mentioned to him that we had to pray for my husband so he would live. He prayed with me, and I told him I had lost my rosary beads that my little granddaughter Kelly had given me. He told me he had a pair in his car and would bring them for me the next time he came to visit. Pastor John brought the rosary beads the next morning. For the next two weeks, he came into my room in the early mornings, and we would pray together.

It was about one week later that a Catholic priest came to see me on a Sunday. I told him about Jean-Pierre, who was still in Sutter Hospital fighting for his life. I asked him if he would be so kind as to go and visit my husband there. He told he would go there and visit him. Later that day in the afternoon, the priest called me and said he had visited Jean-Pierre and prayed with him. I cannot tell you how important prayer is in your life when you have so many odds against you. I know you must stay connected with God on a daily basis with prayers, but I for one had never needed him more in my life than to answer my prayers for my husband's recovery.

I was always two to three weeks further along in recovery than my husband, and I was being moved from one facility to another. His injuries were far worse than mine, but our doctors said he would heal much faster than I would because my recovery would be a long time. They were right because it took me over two and a half years to regain many of my functions like washing my hair with two arms and two hands, and being fully able to dress myself, put on jewelry, comb my hair, and do other tasks that required two hands and two arms to be raised above my shoulders. I have much gratitude to my husband because after he recovered, he helped me more than I ever realized.

My husband's injuries were severe. His left foot and leg went through the floorboard of our truck. The steering wheel crushed his chest, and he had sustained multiple chest, heart, and lung injuries. The entire back of both sides of his lungs were deep purple, black, and dark blue even weeks later when I saw him for the first time in the rehab center. His leg was badly cut to the bone, and it required daily care and cleaning treatments by the nurse. He had been cut from the neck to past his belly button to his pelvic area to reduce the swelling after sustaining two major surgeries in a matter of hours. There was serious concern he would not survive for days and weeks after the accident. After several weeks, there was still concern about the injury to his chest and heart, and there was still blood in his lungs.

Once I was at the nursing home, I finally was able to speak to one of his doctors on the phone. I remember she called me when I was in PT. I asked why it had taken so long for someone to call me about my husband's health status, and she said, "Well, we only speak to one family member, and they are supposed to report to the other family members the status of your husband's health." I discovered the only person they spoke with was my husband's daughter, and since she was with him constantly, she never called me to speak with me about his well-being. I was dumbfounded and requested that my name be placed on his communication board now, after three weeks of hearing nothing! The female doctor informed me that my husband still had blood in his lungs. I asked if he going to be able to live with that, and she said to me, "If we cannot get the blood out of his lungs, he will die." Fear went through my body at that moment, and I wondered if this nightmare was ever going to end for us. After speaking to the doctor, I was able to stay connected with my husband's doctors from then on.

Not long after that, I received my first phone call from my husband. I could hardly believe my ears when I heard his voice. He did not say much, but what he said to me will last me a lifetime. He said, "I saw God. He sat me down, and we had a long talk together." Nothing else was spoken between us, and I wondered about his mental health after hearing his statement but knew in my heart anything could be possible when someone goes through the trauma my husband had experienced.

## Letters to My Husband
While I was in the rehab center, I wrote letters to my husband. These are the only three letters I was able to write to my husband during our absence from each other.

Dear Jean-Pierre                1-12-09

It was so good to hear your voice today. I miss you so much. I pray for your health to improve every night & I say the rosary each day.

Joe has been good about being there for me about my health needs + taking care of our Household bills + things.

I went to rehab today + will learn How to walk c̄ a "Hemi-walker" + will learn How to dress myself with one arm + Hand.

I am so glad we are both strong + will continue to get better each day.

I love you very much & will never stop loving you after all our years together.

Love, Me

*Dear Jean-Pierre*                                    *1-12-09*

*It was so good to hear your voice today. I miss you so much. I pray for your health to improve every night and I say the rosary each day.*

*Joe has been good about being there for me about my health needs and taking care of our household bills and things.*

*I went to rehab today and will learn how to walk with a "hemi-walker" and I will learn how to dress myself with one arm and hand.*

*I am so glad we are both strong and will continue to get better each day. I love you very much and will never stop loving you after all our years together.*

*Love, Me*

To my dear Husband Jean-Pierre,

I pray for your good health to return quickly. I know you are a strong man & will do everything needed ### to get better. I think of you often and miss being near to you, (I miss you)

For me I am improving & now move from Roseville KP to Eskaton Fair Oaks for more time & physical therapy.

We are both so lucky to have family & friends who love us & care so much to help us in all matters. They are all to good to us.

Remember to pray.

I love you forever & always, me

*To My dear Husband Jean-Pierre,*

*I pray for your good health to return quickly. I know you are a strong Man and will do everything needed to get better. I think of you often and miss being near to you. For me I am improving and now move from Roseville KP to Eskaton Fair Oaks for more time with physical therapy.*

*We are both so lucky to have family and friends who love us and care so much to help us with all matters. They are all too good to us. Remember to pray. I love you forever and always, Me*

To My Dear Love: Jean-Pierre

I hope you are feeling better each day. I'am glad to know you are doing well enough to be moved from ICU. I miss you every moment + look forward to the day that I'am allowed to see you soon. I can not wait to go home + be together again.

I'am doing good in Physical therapy each day but very tired too. I'am walking better c̄ a new cane + learning How to do Kitchen work c̄ one here. I must also build up, my strenght before I can go to Joe's house + then il can come to see you too.

Remember I love you so much. + pray for you each night. God Bless you —
Love, me XOXOXOX

*To My Dear Love: Jean-Pierre*

*I hope you are feeling better each day. I am glad to know you are doing well enough to be moved from ICU. I miss you every moment and look forward to the day I am allowed to see you soon. I cannot wait to go home and be together again.*

*I am doing good in physical therapy each day but very tired too. I am walking better with a new cane and learning how to do kitchen work with one hand. I must also build up my strength before I can go to Joe's house and then I can come to see you too. Remember I love you so much and pray for you each night. God Bless you.*

*Love, Me xoxoxox*

## My Husband Coming to Same Rehab Center—Hurray!

After a few weeks, my husband was well enough to be transferred to Kaiser Roseville Hospital. He was put in the telemetry unit, however, because they were still concerned about his heart and lungs. He was there for about a week before I got the news that he was going to join me in the rehab center. The male nurse said to me one bright morning, "Mrs. Korn, I hear Mr. Korn will be coming to our facility tomorrow." It was music to my ears. I could hardly believe it as I made sure I heard him correctly. "Yes, he should be here about noon tomorrow." I could not get over my excitement and joy; my prayers had been answered.

The next day, I decided I had had enough of the paper diapers I was wearing. I did not have one mess in them, and I was not about to meet my husband with a diaper on. I decided to take the paper thing off myself, one-handed or not, and the nursing staff did not need to know about it. I thought it was the first step in the right direction of being in control of me. I made sure to try to look my best the day my husband was to arrive at the hospital. I do not think I had my makeup bag, but I made sure to have my hair combed and to look my best in a hospital gown and wheelchair to greet him.

Noon came and passed, and I was beginning to get very anxious as I double-checked with the nurse to make sure he was coming. I wheeled myself to the long corridor where there were full glass windows as I waited for the hospital van to deliver him. My heart was racing as each vehicle entered the parking lot, and I stared at each hospital van and ambulance to see if it was him. I felt like a school girl waiting on the corner for her boyfriend so she could kiss him before her parents find out. My heart was beating so fast that I could hardly stand it. When three o'clock came and went, I began to feel discouraged but would not give up hope since I kept hearing he was still coming.

I remember being in the hallway of the rehab center close to the nurses' station when I first saw his daughter enter the room, and just behind her came my husband in a wheelchair, sitting up to my amazement! Glory be to God—it was really him. The man I had prayed for every waking hour for weeks was sitting before me. He was completely shaven, his beard and mustache gone, and his head was completely shaved as well. He looked terribly thin, and I had a flash of a holocaust victim, but I knew it was him because of the way he smiled at me.

We said nothing to each other; only our eyes spoke the look of love as we sat in our wheelchairs staring at each other like two lost lovers who had been reunited. We did not have the strength to get up and hug each other. He looked so frail I was fearful to get near him, but he was alive and breathing and sitting right in front of me, even if it was only for a second before they showed him to his room. The rehab center was kind and was trying to place us in the same room together, but there were not enough beds available to do so. Therefore, we were a few doors down from each other for the next couple of days. For the next three days before I was to be released, I now had my husband back under one roof again with me. I could see and visit with him as long as I cared to, and I could be by his side until we both went to sleep. How wonderful.

## Welcome to My World

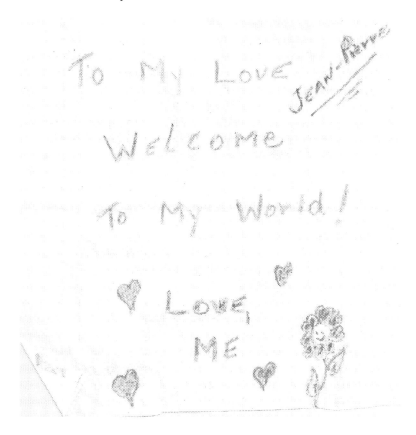

This is the note I placed on Jean-Pierre's room wall when he arrived at the rehab center so he could see it from his bed.

The next day, the PT person came to Jean-Pierre's room and helped him stand next to the bathroom sink to brush his teeth and wash. She held on to him with a special strap or belt to give him support to stand. As the days passed, he was able to go the PT department, and the first exercise they gave him was to hit a yellow balloon back and forth to the PT to determine his strength level. He was able to hit the balloon back and forth for one minute before becoming exhausted. After witnessing this exercise, I knew he had a long way to go, but at least he was standing for one minute and was aware of what was happening around him.

His daughter made sure to bring in lots of rich and fattening foods that he loved in order to keep him eating. He was one of the best-fed persons at the rehab center, but he also needed some nutrition like chicken soup. After Jean-Pierre was at the rehab center for three days, his daughter felt he was in good enough hands to be able to fly back home to South Carolina and return to her business and life again. I was happy that both his daughters had flown out to be with him during a very critical time for him. I knew if anyone could keep him alive and get him to want to keep living, they could do it for him.

In many ways, I was blessed not to have witnessed the critical state he was in those early days. I frankly do not know if I would have made it, seeing him suffer so. Once Jean-Pierre was at the rehab center with me, I was strong enough to make sure he would be well cared for by the nursing staff.

## Out of Rehab: Watch Out, Son, Mom's Moving In!

The reward for my son coming every day to visit me at the rehab center was that when two weeks later I was able to leave, it was his home I moved into so that he could monitor my care and progress. In addition, my husband was still in the rehab center in Sacramento, and with my son living in same city, it would allow me to be able to visit him each day. It was much farther from Cool, and I was nowhere near driving on my own yet.

My son was driving me to my home to retrieve some clothes, and it would be the first time I would be in my home since the accident. On the way there, we were on Highway 193, and I saw a large wooden cross placed exactly where the accident had occurred. It then dawned on me this was a representation of where the man had lost his life. I remember crying out loud by the shock of seeing it there; it was so confirming that someone had lost their life right at that very spot. My son was very patient with me and said it was understandable that I would be upset by seeing it. Every day from that time forward, my husband and I have to be reminded of the accident since the cross is placed so close to our home. Every time we drive from our house and use Highway 193 toward Cool, we witness its presence.

Three days later, I was released from the rehab center and went to stay at my son's for a few weeks. My son Joe had made arrangements for a hospital bed for me to be placed in the middle of his living room. This is exactly where Pooh Bear, his orange cat, warmed himself in the sunlight each day. Pooh Bear was not happy to see that my hospital bed now occupied his warming spot. It was kind of comical when Pooh Bear came home each day, would walk in the house, and take one look at me out of the corner of his eye. He would then give a look as if to say, "You're still here? When are you leaving?" He made me chuckle with his behavior, and I knew he was not fond of me and my big hospital bed.

I received excellent home care from Accent Care Services at my son's home with day nurses to help me shower, a surgical nurse to clean my wounds, and a social worker and PT who came to my son's home to help me get adjusted to my surroundings.

A few days later, I had a dream about my father, who had died several years prior. He was wearing a red Pendleton shirt (he always wore Pendleton shirts in San Francisco, where he lived), and he said to me, "I came to help you. I did not take my Alzheimer's medication today so I could see you." A short time after that, when I was at my son's home alone, the lights began to flicker. I found this to be interesting because the night my mother was dying, and for many nights after her death, the lights would flicker when I was stressed. I took both of these signs to mean my parents were thinking of me and encouraging me to move forward.

# PART III:

## AS TIME GOES BY

*Each of us has to walk in the dark at some time,*
*and it is up to us to turn on the light.*
—Katharine Hepburn

I t was about three weeks into the recovery and healing
process when I was staying with my son that I experienced
a loss of spirit and a loss of self-purpose in my life. Here is my
journey through this dark period and the unexpected happiness
I discovered at the end of it.

### Loss of Spirit and Self-Purpose

While I was staying at my son's home, something came over me
that I had never experienced before. I had lost my spirit. I have
been through some pretty turbulent times in my life, but never
before did I have the sense of not wanting to go forward with my
life. I felt extremely tried, too tired to move forward and keep

trying in life. I felt hollow inside and empty, as if nothing mattered anymore. Things were not improving fast enough for me, and the nightmare of what happened to us just seemed to go on and on at such a slow pace with no end. I had lost all my independence. I had to rely on others to take me places, and I had no choice in how long it would take my body to recover, if ever.

I felt lost, and my spirit was gone. This frightened me because I'm one who has a tremendous energy to fight, but now all the fight was gone. I remember telling my son I had lost my spirit in hopes of some response from him that would encourage me to move forward, but he was at a loss for words. I do not know if it happened when I had to ask my eleven-year-old granddaughter if she would help me get dressed in the morning and help me undress at night. With the use of only one arm, I could not get my bra on or off. We were in her bedroom, and she responded with, "I do not know how to do it." I said to her, "I will tell you how." I felt so awful having to ask a small child to help me get dressed and undressed.

I was in a deep depression and wondered if I would ever regain my spirit—and if I did, how long would it take? Along with losing my spirit, I also lost my sense of purpose in life. What was I good for anymore anyway? I felt completely useless, and my sense of purpose no longer existed from within. I used to take care of my large house, but washing all the floors, doing all the laundry, shopping for groceries, cooking meals, opening the mail, and driving a car were all impossible tasks for me now. I could not even write a personal check to pay my bills on my own. The pleasure of working in my garden—planting flowers, pulling weeds, using the weed-eater, and shoveling dirt—was gone. I could not even wash myself or wash my hair without assistance. I could not perform any task without the help and assistance of someone else. Yes, I had lost my sense of purpose, and along with it, I lost my spirit.

## Psychological Therapy: The Art of Positive Thinking

Being in my sixties, I thought I knew myself pretty well, but experiencing a significant emotional event can cause havoc with your mind, body, and spirit. In addition to losing my spirit and my purpose in my life, I was having flashbacks, seeing those headlights come crashing in on us and not being able to move. It gave me a feeling of helplessness and a sense of worthlessness, as well as terrible nightmares and an ongoing fear that life would never be the same again. The only thing I could hold on to and cling to for myself was prayer and pleading and bartering with God to make it all better again.

I'm thankful for the professionals in the psychiatric fields who helped me and my husband pass through this dark period in our lives to regain a sense of self again. It is good to know that with good work and practice, many of us can get out of a deep depression and become instrumental in dealing with our own post-traumatic stress symptoms. We can work through the pain and anguish to become the person we were meant to be.

I had post-traumatic stress disorder (PTSD) after the car accident. Some of the symptoms I was experiencing included flashbacks, nightmares, and sleep disturbances. I made an appointment to see a psychiatrist, and she said I was very lucky because she had never had an appointment with someone who had survived a head-on car accident. She said most of her visits were to comfort the family members because the person had died.

Since I had been experiencing nightmares and flashbacks, she recommended I see a psychological therapist. This advice turned out to be very helpful. One of the tools the therapist provided was to change my negative thoughts to positive thinking. I was instructed to think of something positive every time my mind went into a negative mode. For example: when I would have thoughts of the car accident, instead of dwelling on the accident, I was told to think about the fact that I had survived the accident. I tried this method several times and found it to be useful in changing my thought process from negative thinking to positive thinking. I found it to be comforting, and I have used this method many times whenever I have had a negative thought. When I changed my way of thinking to a more positive outlook, I experienced fewer flashbacks and negative thoughts about the accident.

Now more than three years later, I do not think as often about the accident unless I'm driving in similar weather conditions, such as a foggy day or night, or when a careless driver drives too fast around me and passes me over a double line. When a driver drives carelessly around me, I tend to get very frightened and sometimes panic. When someone on the opposite side of the road is passing another car, and it is racing toward me, again I become very fearful and tend to slow down to see if they are going to get back into their lane again safely. I have to work on relaxing myself at times like this so that I do not panic.

## Artwork: Healing the Inner You

My husband's doctor had recommended oil painting because he could sit down while doing it, and it also help kept his mind off his weakness and being on oxygen all the time. He wanted to paint three oil paintings, one for each of his daughters as a thank-you for caring for him while he was in the hospital. When we both went to the art store to purchase some supplies, it all became too much for him, and he became exhausted and had to sit down, so we immediately went home for him to rest. The little episode in the art store was enough for me to realize he really was not strong enough to do anything but go to the doctors' appointments.

However, once we got home, he recovered and began to set up an art studio in our home. It was very good for him, and it did help him forget his discomfort and pain. He concentrated on his paintings and how each picture would be made especially for each daughter. One daughter loves castles, so he did an oil painting of a famous castle in Germany for her. He used bright, cheerful colors to reflect his interpretation of the castle. The other two paintings were of landscapes and water scenes.

As he began his paintings, he was so quiet and involved in his work. It almost seemed like our life was back to normal when he was painting and doing what he loved again. It seemed to be healing for his inner spirit.

## Pet Therapy

One year before the accident, I joined a pet-therapy class to learn more about this interesting theory of pets helping patients heal and to discover the love and warmth an animal can provide to the patient. In 2006, we purchased a beautiful yellow lab we named Togo. He was just a puppy, and we gave him all our love and attention as we introduced him to his new home and surroundings, As he began to grow, we taught him all the basic commands for dog manners and obedience. However, it was my hope for Togo to one day become a pet-therapy dog so that we could go visit patients in the hospital and bring some light and happiness into their day. Little did I know that I would someday be one of those patients and in need of some doggy love, kindness, and attention myself.

Once we were home from the rehab center, Togo returned to our house after a long, unexpected visit to our nephew and niece's house. Thank God they rescued him from the kennel the night the accident happened. We had not been able to return home for over one month. I shiver to think of what might have happened to him if he would have been left unattended and forgotten. Again, thank God for family members who step up to plate to help out.

The love and comfort Togo provided to us during our healing process is immeasurable. He had not forgotten us and sat by our side and licked our wounds and bandages. He knew instinctively that we were hurting. As time went on and I began to use a cane, with Togo on a leash, we would take slow walks together around our property. He knew instinctively that I could not walk fast anymore and that each step was a process for me to achieve. He loved working with me and enjoyed every moment of the slow and steady pace it took to recover in the walking process. As time went on, Togo would walk with me to the mailbox and carry the mail home in a pouch bag placed under his neck. He loved getting a dog cookie at the end of the trail for his good behavior and work.

We have all heard of the dog that will fetch your newspaper and slippers for you. Well, Togo is excellent for finding our shoes or slippers around the house and bringing them to us as we sit in our armchairs, saving our strength. As time went on, Togo was trained to wear a harness and pull my garden cart or red wagon with garden equipment, supplies, and tools around the property with me. He will patiently wait when we have reached our destination and relax and lie down until I'm ready to move on. When I go swimming, he patiently waits by the pool and relaxes under a large shade tree. When I'm ready to go back into the house, he escorts me back and waits while I dry myself off. When my husband gets up in the morning, Togo is always there to greet him. When my husband goes to let him out in the morning, if he forgets to turn off the house alarm, Togo will stand near the alarm area to remind him to first turn it off.

The love, time, and devotion Togo has provided me has won him the true title of my best friend. He lets me know when someone has arrived at our gate, or when an animal has trespassed on our property, and then he sleeps where he can keep an eye on me and be ready for protect me at a moment's notice. His love and licks are always there to show me how much he cares, and it warms my heart and heals my soul.

Another type of comfort for the suddenly disabled when you cannot get around much and are in the recovery process is bird watching. I have a small back patio for viewing. I have placed a bird feeder there, and I scatter wild bird seed on the patio stones for those birds that are too timid to use the feeder. This is wonderful entertainment, and the birds put on quite a show for you.

You can view them in their natural environment and discover all the wonders of the different species. I have found great comfort in bird watching, and it is a wonderful way to pass the time when you are homebound.

## We Are Back Home: Home Sweet Home

Coming home again was both exciting and scary. I was thrilled Jean-Pierre and I would be coming home together. I was being driven home by my son, and Jean-Pierre arrived by convalescent car to our home. Our niece was at the home to greet us. She was a tremendous help in making sure the house was in order during our hospital stays and that the plants were cared for as well as our dog.

So on February 2, 2009, I walked into my home again to reclaim it. Jean-Pierre went into the house on a gurney. Our niece had been there for the arrival of his hospital bed and oxygen tanks. The entire living room had been converted into a hospital room for him. He had everything he needed to be bedridden with all medications, hospital supply needs, and TV trays at his bedside. In the back area on a table in the living room were all his medications, wound-care supplies, bedclothes, and grooming needs for easy access. Since I would be unable to go upstairs to our bedroom to retrieve these items, everything he needed was in one room for him. We were instructed by the company's representative on how to use the oxygen tanks and how much oxygen to administer for my husband's comfort level. For the time being, I was going to use our guest bedroom downstairs so that I could be close to Jean-Pierre at a moment's notice.

When we were all settled in the home, Patricia, our other niece, came to spend the first night with us. She prepared our dinner, and we were grateful to have her with us for the first night at home. The next day, my cousin Kathy came from the Petaluma area to help out for a few days. I was so thankful for all the support and assistance we were receiving from our loved ones.

Just as Kathy was driving up our driveway, she discovered fire engines there at our home. We had spent only one night in our home when Jean-Pierre was experiencing difficulty breathing and was in extreme discomfort, He was experiencing chest pain, or as he described it, "Like an elephant sitting on my chest." I called 911, and the Cool Fire Department came once again to our rescue. They made a quick decision to transport Jean-Pierre by ambulance to the nearest hospital.

Kathy had a look of confusion on her face when she arrived after a three-hour drive to see us. She found herself turning around and leaving with me to see what was wrong with Jean-Pierre. This new episode threw me into a panic, and I began to worry about whether he was ready to come home after all. Not knowing which hospital they took Jean-Pierre to, we drove to Roseville Sutter Hospital. They informed us he was not there but did try to locate where he was. We discovered he had been taken to Auburn Faith Hospital, which was much closer to our home than Roseville. So there we were chasing ambulances and trying to get to Jean-Pierre as soon as possible.

He was held under observation for several hours. They finally released him to us and let him go home with us. The doctors felt he may have had a panic attack and needed his oxygen adjusted. They gave him some instructions: "Take a deep breath and get up and move around. When on oxygen, you can get short of breath with this type of injury to the lungs. Breathe slowly through your nose. Give it time to go into the lungs, and get as deep a breath as you can to go into the lungs. Three or four times a day, walk until you're a little tried and coordinate your breathing with walking, but do not wait until you are exhausted. Every five or ten feet, stop and breathe without walking, and do not get short of breath. Coordinate breathing with your exercise. It is not a bad thing to go to bed and rest. Work with what makes you most anxious; it takes some practice to do. It was very unlikely a serious problem, and this type of thing usually happens early on. Use the spirometer to expand your lungs every hour. Gentle, deep breaths are very important."

We got him home, settled him down, and reassured him everything was going to be okay. In time, he began to use his wheelchair and walker, but it proved to be problematic because the oxygen cord was constantly getting tangled up with his walker or wheelchair. I also discovered Jean-Pierre was experiencing night terrors and thinking about the fear of driving in the fog, fear of driving at night, and the flashbacks of the other car's highlights. These thoughts could also contribute to his problems with breathing comfortably while on oxygen.

Kathy was a great help in cooking for us and taking care of our immediate needs. After a few days, she went home, and my brother Anthony came up from Danville to take over and assist us in our daily living needs. It was wonderful to have our family members give so much of their selves to help us get adjusted to our home again. I remember Anthony helping me wrap up

Christmas presents that still needed to be delivered by mail, and we were in the month of February. One does not fully realize the value of family members and loved ones who give so unselfishly of themselves to help others when one cannot do for him or herself.

On February 4, 2009, we saw Jean-Pierre's doctor as a follow up to his emergency visit to Auburn Faith Hospital. I wrote a letter to his doctor requesting home care services.

*Jean-Pierre's Eskaton Care Center discharge papers state all activities he is to have supervision and assistance: showering, walking with the walker, and dressing, transferring from bed to wheelchair, and transferring from a car.*

*Since he has been home (Monday, Feb. 2, 2009), he has only a limited amount of family members to be able to help him on a full-day basis. We will only have family help until Feb. 8, 2009. I'm unable to provide assistance, and he often does not take my advice regarding supervision. Last night he decided to take a shower on his own although we have a shower chair, and I'm the only one available to assist him. I was exhausted because we had just returned after six hours at Auburn Faith Hospital due to his having shortness of breath and trembling with chills.*

*Here is what happened at 1:00 p.m., February 3, 2009. I took his blood pressure, and it was 120/83. Therefore, Jean-Pierre felt it was okay to take his medications. Within twenty minutes, his coloring changed to a dull gray and he was having difficulty breathing. I took his blood pressure again, and it was 104/93. I turned his oxygen level up from 2 to 3. I then called 911, and the medics arrived and took him to Auburn Faith Hospital via ambulance. He saw a* doctor, and the doctor did not know what happened. After six long hours, he was released to go home again.

I have seven pins in my forearm and a permanent rod and screw in my upper arm. I was completely exhausted with only four pain pills (which were not working) and no food for hours. My lower back was in spasms and hurts terribly when I'm up too long and trying to care for his needs. I was unable to do my own exercises, without food, or get my own rest due to this incident. By the time I got home and helped him with his bath and all the other needs for him, I was moved to tears and my own B/P was 190/114.

Therefore, since I'm unable to provide adequate care for him, I'm requesting some nursing assistance and supervision as much as possible for my husband. This way he will not only be doing what is right in progressing and improving, but also my own health will not be jeopardized. He is high maintenance due to his multiple health issues and can have the tendency to be very needy. It is just too much for me alone to provide for him because I'm just too weak, too sick, and in pain.

## Home Care Services

Jean-Pierre's doctor approved many different services to help us get through the recovery period at home. We both had nurse's aides to help us bathe, physical therapists to show us exercises for each step of the recovery process, surgical nurses to change and clean our surgery sites, and I had an occupational therapist to help me with daily activities using one arm. These professionals are worth their weight in gold, and we came to look forward to seeing them as many as four times a week. They not only helped us regain our confidence, but also provided hope that better days were ahead for us. They truly cared about helping us improve our situations and offered many suggestions and recommendations for a faster recovery period. We quickly became true allies working together for a common cause.

I felt cared for and valued by these wonderful people. Even the oxygen service delivery man was helpful by being friendly when resupplying my husband's oxygen tanks. He told us about another delivery that he went to on our route that involved an entire family of five in another horrible head-on car accident where one fifteen-year-old girl had lost both legs. We thought about how lucky we were to be recovering with all our limbs intact and how awful it was for the young girl who had lost her legs. He had mentioned how the entire family was placed in hospital beds at their home and how so many care providers were there all the time to help this family recover.

As for me, I have always been a very independent person. I have done everything for myself from a very early age. In fact, the only one I could ever depend on was myself, so it was very hard to have my life change to where I needed friends and family to help me with every part of my life. Along with the nurses, doctors, and care providers whom I heavily depended on to help me get through the immediate recovery phase, there was home care from the many care providers who did a wonderful job assisting me to become a whole person again. I cannot say enough wonderful things about these very devoted people who have made this their life profession. They are the thankless group where everyone just expects them to do their job and make us better, but there is another factor to consider, and that is up to me. It is up to me to do my part in making myself better by working through the pain and becoming all I can be. I owe it to myself to take the bull by the horns and say, "I can do this. I know I can, and if I cannot do it today, I will be able to do it tomorrow."

## The First Year of Recovery

The first year of recovery was both frustrating and rewarding. Frustration occurs when you have to rely on everyone else to do the simple, easy things you took for granted before your disability, such as cutting your own meat on your plate, preparing your own meals, and taking a bath or using the toilet by yourself. These simple tasks we all take for granted have now become major ordeals to deal with in day-to-day activities. It is easy for one to say, "Be patient. Everything is going to get better," but living through this period hour after hour and day after day can wear on anyone's nerves and frustration level. The good news is that time is a great healer. If you follow doctors' orders and do your physical therapy exercises religiously, things will improve. I soon discovered that what I could not do one or two months before, I could now master, and I looked forward to continued progress.

It was still winter when the doctor decided it was time to remove the seven pins in my wrist and arm. His nurse called me for an appointment to have them removed, and I requested some pain medication to be administered before removing them in his office. She informed me that was not necessary because even five-year-old children did not need medication to remove their pins. On that day, I entered the doctor's examination room feeling nervous and scared about the possibility of experiencing more pain with the removal of the pins.

When the doctor removed the smaller pins from my wrists and lower arm areas, it did not seem too painful, and I was somewhat relieved. However, when he began to remove the larger pins, which looked more like nails, the removal was excruciating. At one point, the doctor was pulling with all his might and with great force. I do not know if it was the size of the pins or the bones moving back into position, but it took all I could not to scream in pain. I remember looking over at the medical assistant who told me it would not hurt and wanting to choke her, if only I had two hands to do it with. I had questions for the doctor but could not even gather my thoughts due to the pain I was experiencing. I remember leaving the examination room as soon as I could and going to the nearest ladies room to find a stall and cry my eyes out from the pain. This pain continued from the time of the appointment for removal, which was at about 10:30 a.m., until 9:00 that night, even after taking medication to stop the pain. What an ordeal that was, one I hope never to experience again.

## Spring 2009

In March, we purchased a new 2009 tan GMC truck out of necessity because we didn't have a vehicle for transportation. For the first month home, we had to depend on family members to take us to all our medical and physical therapy appointments. We used the truck only for necessary appointments and groceries. At this time, we did not want to travel by car or truck at all because it was too emotional for us.

In April, my husband was able to get off the oxygen on a twenty-four-hour basis. I was so pleased we had made another accomplishment in his recovery period. April was also the month we both were able to climb up sixteen steps from our downstairs to our bedroom and finally sleep in our own bed. It felt so wonderful to hold hands with each other and take each step slowly as we climbed the staircase. When we got to the top of the stairwell, I breathed a sigh of relief. We made it to our bedroom together! We also started to take our whirlpool tub baths together to help each other bathe. I would help him when he was too tired, and he would help me when I needed help getting into and out of the tub. There was my husband, a man who was sixty-nine and never had a scar on his body prior to the accident. Now he was a mass of scars on his torso and legs. It was difficult to view them and see what torture he had overcome. Gradually, I got used to seeing his mass of scars on his torso, and using my positive thinking skills, I was just thankful he was alive and beginning to get well again. The whirlpool baths were wonderful for all our sore muscles and limbs. For our safety, we put hand-grip bars on the bathtub area for easily getting in and out of the tub. A long-handle scrub brush was helpful in reaching areas that were now too difficult to do with our own hands.

It was on April 26, 2009, when we had a Celebration of Life party and a thank-you for the fire departments' rescue teams and all the other special people who helped us so much during our recovery period. It was also at that time that I finally was able to find some peace regarding the man who lost his life at the scene of our car accident. I told the psychiatrist I was seeing that we were planning a Celebration of Life party for my husband and me but that I felt guilty about the man who had lost his life. Her suggestion was before the day of the celebration to have a quiet moment with myself and write a letter to the man who had passed, expressing my feelings for him and his loss of life. I did just that the day before our celebration. I wrote a letter and placed in our wishing well, which is placed close to his property line where he was living. I also placed a candle and some flowers in the wishing well as a final good-bye and held a private ceremony in his honor. This action was very helpful to me, and I found peace by holding a private ceremony for him and letting him know I cared about his life and was sorry for what happened.

When the time came for the fire departments' rescue teams to come and join us for the celebration, they arrived in their fire trucks and chief's car. This was a wonderful statement for all our guests and family and friends. Everyone had a good time with good food and music, and I planned a small ceremony and thank-you gifts for each fire department and Danielle, the lady who was the first to show up at our rescue. She also came with her mother. I was so pleased; everything turned out beautifully. Jean-Pierre presented each of his paintings to his daughters, and the pictures turned out really nice. At the end of the party, everyone released colorful balloons in the sky to make a wish on. The entire sky above our house was filled with beautiful red, white, green, blue, pink, and yellow balloons reaching for the heavens.

It was May 2009 when it occurred to me while driving our truck that I was holding a cup of coffee with my left hand. What an accomplishment for me. I was so proud that I could finally lift a cup of coffee with my left hand.

## Summer 2009

In July 2009, we had a swimming pool built for us in our backyard. It looked beautiful and so inviting. I was thrilled that I could add to my physical therapy treatments with swimming every day in the summer. Life was starting to look up again even if I struggled with reaching out to make a swimming stroke. By the end of summer, I was swimming nine hundred strokes within one half hour. Wow, this was progress. Swimming is a great sport because you become weightless in the water, and it becomes much easier to move about in the water.

On July 9, 2009, my sister Sandra died from breast cancer. She had refused to get chemotherapy or any treatments for her disease. I had made efforts to see her, but she refused to see me due to the estranged relationship we had for several years. Honoring and respecting her request, it was difficult to know that the next time I would see her would be in her coffin. These are the mistakes and regrets we make in life, and I have to live with it for eternity.

In September 2009, we celebrated Jean-Pierre's seventieth

birthday with friends and family at the poolside, blessing it with a bottle of champagne. We also had a wonderful party and celebrated my husband's being off oxygen for several months now and being able to have fun with family and friends.

It was summer when I wrote a letter to my doctor explaining some of the difficulty I was still experiencing:

*Regarding my left arm, every day I experience multiple sites of pain in my left arm. There is pain traveling along the side of the outer edge of my left forearm.*

*I cannot go to sleep at night without sleep medication.*

*I cannot get into a comfortable position in bed because this is the arm I usually sleep on when on my side.*

*I still have very little strength in this arm for lifting items.*

*I can be doing nothing, and it will create pain for me.*

*If I try to do housework like sweeping and dressing myself, on the left side, using my arm is terribly painful. I'm unable to do most chores that require repetition.*

*There are many things I still am unable to do.*

*What is the cause of the pain? How long will I have to endure the pain?*

*I'm now getting pain in the right hand near the wrist and the thumb area.*

*Is my arm still broken in the upper area?*

*I still have swelling in my left hand and fingers.*

*I'm unable to make a closed fist.*

## Additional Surgeries

As the months passed, I continued to experience pain in the upper left arm where the rod had been placed and down in the lower part of my arm. I decided to go see my doctor to discover what was going on. My arm felt like there was a huge, hard baseball placed in my upper arm, and even if I used ice packs or hot pads, nothing seemed to relieve the pain I was experiencing. After my doctor took X-rays of my injured arm, he informed me the bone had not grown back together again and it should have by now. Instead of growing together, it was growing in an outward position, and nerve pain from the rod could be the reason for the pain I was experiencing in my lower arm.

My doctor recommended removal of the rod and to replace it with a plate and screws to help relieve the pain I was still experiencing. I was not excited about a second surgery, but I could not continue to live with the pain in my lower arm either, so the decision was made to have surgery in November 2009 to remove the rod and replace it with a plate and screws. The doctor also thought I needed to take a piece of bone from my pelvis and place it in the area where the upper arm bone was not growing together.

I didn't want to think about more surgeries when the first one was already more than I could handle. However, the real picture is there are times when we have to endure more surgeries in order to find comfort and function to the fullest extent. I experienced four surgeries in two years. The worst part of this process was the recovery period and trying to regain my strength and health again.

Instead of being a couch potato who gets comfortable wearing bedclothes all day and sitting in front of the television, I had to work hard at becoming whole again and adding meaning to my life. I learned that each surgery is different from the last one. Thinking it is all going to be easy and better than the last one is very optimistic, but some things never go as planned. I needed to be psyched up for the next surgery to give it my best. I had to sustain a positive mental attitude and know in my heart of hearts this too would pass and I would get better.

## The Second Surgery

*I just received a phone message from the surgery scheduler nurse. My second surgery is confirmed for November 19, 2009. My stomach does not feel very well right now because as I mark the calendar for the date, I now realize this is for real. I'm now going to have a recorrective surgery on my upper arm. My fears are I only want to survive the anesthesia. I know I can handle the recovery period with the pain and all. I do not like to take pain medication or sleeping pills but now realize that I will have to take them for a second round. I worked really hard at getting off them the first time, and I had some withdrawals but was surprised the sleeping pills were relatively easy to get off. To get to sleep on my own was not as bad as I thought it would be. I guess I will be going back to physical therapy again.*

*I'm determined to regain the strength and function in my left arm. I want to be able to perform all the functions I did prior to the car accident. My doctor states in time I will be able to do housework and return to gardening again without experiencing pain. He feels the pain is being caused by nerve pressure from the rod that is placed in my upper arm. I sure hope he is correct. I would love to return to doing full-house cleaning and using the weed-eater in all my gardens that surround my home. I want to feel useful, and I want to live a full life well into my old age. Well, it looks like there will be a new chapter in my left arm regarding a second surgery.*

In many ways, my experience with the second surgery was more difficult for me to endure. I do not know if it was because there was a second surgery at the same site or that I was not on as much pain medication. All I know is that it was a grueling recovery. This time, instead of small incisions, I had a long incision that went down two-thirds of my left upper arm with many metal staples. The swelling and pain were almost intolerable. I would try everything to help the pain go away. After I was home, my arm was propped up on pillows as I was lying on my back, and multiple ice packs were applied throughout the day, but little helped to ease the suffering.

Jean-Pierre was wonderful and very attentive to me, but I was in terrible pain most of my waking hours. I had sleeping pills to help me get much-needed rest but then would have terrible nightmares. I remember feeling like I just wanted to die because it seemed like the pain would never get better and it was now almost one year from the first surgery.

My husband came to my bedside one night after a horrible nightmare about grease and filth covering me and the entire inside of my home. He tried to comfort me, as I was in tears and exhausted. As he leaned on my bed rail, he said, "It's going to be okay. Look forward to the spring time, and all the flower bulbs you planted will be coming up, and they will look so pretty." It helped me to think that there were brighter days ahead, and I thanked him for his kind words. I frankly do not know what I would have done without my husband by my side and loving me so much.

## The Third Surgery

In December, with the many metal staples still intact in my upper arm, I was scheduled for another surgery. This time, my mammogram showed questionable sites of tumors in my breasts. We were all hopeful that the tumors were from the trauma of the seatbelt injuries, but since the needle biopsies failed, the surgeon could not be certain. Due to the strong history of breast cancer in my family, it was considered wise to undergo breast biopsies on December 4, 2009. There were multiple tumors, but only two were most concerning to my surgeon. The one bright thought was that while under anesthesia, the surgeon could also remove the metal staples in my arm at the same time.

I was happy to be informed it was not cancer but injury and trauma from the seatbelts that caused the oil-based tumors. One breast biopsy site got infected, and I had many follow-up care appointments to clean the wound that left a deep scar over my breast. The surgeon said I was ready for a break and he was glad it was not breast cancer, but follow-up mammograms would be required for the next several years. Actually, I do not think I could have tolerated any more bad news, so I was very relieved to not have breast cancer too.

Recovering from the breast biopsies, I discovered it was pretty painful to sleep at night where the surgery sites were located. I found that wearing a sleeping bra helped with easing the pain in that area. I wore the sleeping bras to bed for weeks and would recommend that to anyone who experiences the discomfort of breast biopsies. I have continued to use the sleeping bras in my waking hours due to the comfort and ability to slip them over my head without having to use two arms to put them on with hooks and eyes.

While I was recovering from surgery and healing, I was in need of much assistance. My husband was there for me every step of the way. Jean-Pierre was wonderful in helping through all my daily activities by helping me get dressed and undressed, cutting my meat and food at all meals, and providing assistance with bathing and hair washing. In addition, he was doing most of the daily house chores, and it was then we decided we needed a housekeeper and gardener to help with the majority of the work around the house and the property.

By this time, my right arm and shoulder were getting very tired of doing the work for two arms for a long time. I was beginning to have pain in my right shoulder, and it was becoming increasingly difficult to raise my right arm over my head to reach for dishes in the cabinet and any other items that required reaching above my head, such as washing and combing my hair. It got to the point I could no longer reach with my right arm above my eye level.

The good news was my left arm began to heal from the second surgery. I no longer experienced the pain I had prior to surgery in my lower arm. That was good news for me; at least one area was free of pain. I now had to concentrate on strength building and focus on physical therapy to get my left arm as back to normal as possible. I knew this would take time and full concentration on my part, and I was determined to never give up on my physical therapy exercises.

## Still Recovering

I happened to come across an old note that I had brought with me to a doctor's visit in reference to what I still could not do one year after my second surgery. Everything takes time, and sometimes we have to work really hard for improvement to happen. In my case, if I wanted to have full use of my arms, I had to overcome the following list of things I still could not do two years since the accident.

*Concerns I have about my ability to use my arms. With or without pain, my arm catches me off guard. This creates anxiety in me in the following:*

*Cannot lift a large pot of water.*
*Cannot lift a full dinner plate or clear table of a stack of plates.*
*Cannot lift casserole bowls from oven to counter.*
*Cannot take off clothes or underclothes over head or button up at neck or unbutton at neck.*

*Need help from husband to undress or dress with clothes that require pulling over head.*

*Caught off guard when attempting to put arm around waist of my son for photo—it was very painful.*

*Unable to hang up clothes on clothes rack. Still cannot reach above head to hang clothes.*

*Unable to lift laundry basket from one area to the next area.*

*Have to bring a small chair with wheels in order to move small boxes from one area to another.*

*Drop the telephone when handed to me.*

*All of this makes my good arm worse. It is still painful and limited in reaching above. My right will only reach to my eye level. It is frozen from this point.*

*Past three weeks, husband had to go to ER due to palpitations. He gets lightheaded and/or dizzy, and I am unable to help him due to limitations of pain in arms and limited strength.*

*I'm unable to get out of driveway of my house when trying to drive truck.*

*I'm unable to get used to truck driving for strength that is needed to recorrect. If I turn the wheel hard, it is painful.*

*Basically a one-arm person who lives in a rural area and unable to help my husband when he is ill and needs medical attention. I'm concerned about needing to relocate from Highway 49 if I do not improve. Do not have the physical ability to help my husband to and from the car or truck when he is feeling ill.*

After typing this list of notes of all my disabilities, I can now say, two years later, I have accomplished most of these tasks with or without pain and stiffness when reaching above my head. One of the most important aspects is I'm now able to fully dress and undress myself. It is seldom that I need help to pull a piece of clothing over my head. I now realize I can do these tasks but that my hair will be a mess because I now have to pull the article of clothing over my head instead of raising it above my head and hair. I'm still a little scared to try carrying heavy items from the oven or to the oven, such as a large roast or casserole dish.

I continued to do physical therapy exercises every day to improve the strength in my left arm. I was still going to physical therapy two or three times a week to learn more about what I could do to improve the mobility and strength of my left arm. I was still performing many tasks with just my right arm, and it was beginning to hurt and freeze up on me from overuse. It came to a point where if I needed strength at waist level, I would use my right arm, and if I needed to reach above my head to obtain a dish or glass, I would use my left arm and hand.

As time went on, it was inevitable that I would need another surgery to repair the reaching ability in my overused right arm. It had been doing the work of two arms for two years.

## The Fourth and Final Surgery

On October 20, 2010, I underwent another surgery, now on my right arm. This was the fourth and final surgery that needed to take place in order to put this whole ordeal behind me and to move forward.

Needless to say, after four surgeries in two years, this surgery was much easier than the other two surgeries performed on my left arm. However, following the doctor's orders for a good recovery, I needed to do physical therapy exercises on both arms now. It is very difficult to have multiple surgeries in a short period of time due to the strength it drains you of and the sheer exhaustion of trying to recover. I was getting used to just sitting in my armchair when I was not doing my physical therapy and knew this type of behavior would have to stop. It just seemed like every time I tried to advance myself, another surgery would rear its ugly head, and I would be back at a starting point again.

My doctor had informed me that the year 2011 would be a very good year for me, and he was right. The year 2011 gave me hope that soon all of these surgeries would be put behind me and I could at long last move forward and get on with my life.

When I look back, I remember being in my fifties and not being able to accept how I looked and who I was. I can say now, in my sixties, I have finally accepted myself. I think the sixties will be better for me than the forties and fifties. Even though I started my sixties with a horrible car accident, I have faith that my sixties will be some of the best years of my life. I finally know who I am, and I accept myself and how I look now. I want to still see a lot about life and experience pretty much all there is to life as well. I'm no longer as much of a risk taker as I was before in my younger days. I now know the value of life and how it can be taken away from you in an instant. I'm thankful God has given me a second chance in life to love my husband, family, and friends. I still want to live life to the fullest but know it is up to me if I want that to happen. It means eating right and healthy, exercising, and being mindful to be safe with myself and to be forever grateful for my relationship with my husband. He has been a great support system throughout this terrible ordeal. He gives me strength and believes in me when I'm in doubt about myself.

## The Beauty of Christmas

My niece Tina came over Christmas of 2010 and decorated our home for us. She brought out all our decorations, and the Christmas season had arrived by the time she left our home a few days later. I was so pleased because I love to decorate for the holidays, and with both arms still healing and the breast biopsy sites still painful, I was very grateful for her help. I paid the daughter of my real estate agent to come and wrap Christmas presents for me. She was about twelve and wanted very much to please me and do the job right as I explained how to apply the tissue paper and wrapping paper and place the ribbons. I paid her two dollars a box, and she was able to have some extra Christmas money that year for spending. I made an attempt to wrap some gifts with one arm but decided it was far too frustrating and made the decision to give prepaid gift cards to all those that I did not have a gift for yet. This was the simplest way to celebrate Christmas and be problem-free.

My brother Anthony came over again during the Christmas season and put the lights on the tree and on the outside of the house. I thought this was really nice of both him and Tina to care so much about bringing Christmas to our house.

On New Year's 2011, we were happy to be home and snug in our beds. In my heart and head, I knew it would be a better year for us.

## Traveling: We Are on the Go Again

Almost one year after our accident, we tried our hands at traveling abroad again. I remember going to Europe in May 2010 about six months after my last surgery. I was still healing from the surgery and was uncomfortable at times but tried very hard to think about other things and not let the pain get to me.

No more running after trains to catch while carrying a backpack. Now I travel with a walking cane because I tend to get tired walking long distances, and it helps with my balance. The most trouble we have with traveling is walking with our luggage and standing in long lines. Now, for us, slow and easy wins the race. We just give ourselves enough time to make all our scheduled planes and trains.

Recently, when traveling on an extended vacation, I purchased a flexible folding cane. I found it to be very comfortable, with a softer rubber cushion for my hand and wrists when using it for a long period of time. It was reasonably priced at about twenty dollars, and it could be folded and packed in a backpack when not in use.

In addition, I purchased a suitcase with wheels and an added benefit of a folding-down seat to be used when waiting in long lines where there are no seats available. The seat holds up to three hundred pounds and is very comfortable and stable. It is an expensive purchase of $150, but it has come in handy when needing a seat or chair and there is none to be found. It is a very handsome piece of luggage and very well built with wheels that turn all ways, and it has plenty of room for my laptop and fits all the standard airline dimensions for carrying onboard. It is disability items like these that make life a whole lot easier and help us join the healthy world again.

Taking time to rest is a must when traveling for days on end. When traveling to Machu Picchu, I went for the trip of a lifetime. When we finally arrived at the site after spending much of the morning to get there by bus and train, I was extremely tired. I knew in my heart I could not go much further. The tour guide mentioned the tour would be another three hours on the steep rocky cliff, so I decided to stay and sit on a wooden bench overlooking the beautiful site of Machu Picchu while the others went on and heard all the stories of this magical site. I was not depressed by everyone going off and leaving me behind because I used my positive thinking and was just pleased I had made it this far. I enjoyed talking to other tourists who stopped to rest for a while and visit. When I was alone on the bench, I continued to gaze at the beautiful site and think about all the people who had once lived there and made this place their home. I admired the tourists who took on the mountain peak and looked like little ants from below where I was sitting. No, I did not envy them; I was just glad to have made the trip and to keep the memories for a lifetime.

*I'm only one, but still I am one. I cannot do everything, but still I can do something. I will not refuse to do the something I can do.*

*—Helen Keller*

# Conclusion

## What You Give Up and What You Gain

One of the significant health issues my husband is experiencing is atrial fibrillation. The doctors feel it may or may not be caused by the car accident. I can only say he did not have this problem before the accident. He now takes heart medication to keep his atrial fibrillation under control. Atrial fibrillation is many pulses that may be released at a rapid, unorganized rate. At first, these rapid pulses were very concerning and troubling to my husband, but after visits to the emergency room and doctors' offices, over time my husband has learned to understand and try to relax when these palpations occur. The heart medication has been very effective in reducing these occurrences.

Probably the most significant thing I can say my husband and I have given up is the thrill of taking pleasure trips by driving in the car. Night time is the worst time for us to drive our car or truck because we are fearful of the late-night drivers who may be taking a risk drinking and driving. I used to love to drive my car and take long driving trips at night with the windows down and the cool wind blowing through my hair, or traveling to places where I have never been. Nowadays when we travel, it is mostly during the day and during the weekdays when others are at work. We select when it is important enough to get into our vehicles and risk driving at night. Freeway driving does not bother me as much as driving the highways and two-lane roads. Although the probability of another head-on car accident is almost nil, the fear is impregnated in my mind forever.

Although we have talked about taking a road trip this summer to Yellowstone Park, we have yet to say we are actually going to do it. It is my hope this trip would help us overcome the fear of driving long distances again. I would love to enjoy driving again.

As time and aging catches up with you, learning to give up things you once did with ease becomes a reality. No, I cannot run anymore due to aging, and, yes, my full-body strength is put to the test every time I try to do something I used to do before the accident, such as digging a hole with a shovel or performing any function in excess of three hours. I find if I work in the garden for three hours, it is pretty much my max because pushing beyond that point, I run the risk of hurting or falling due to exhaustion. But I can now pull weeds with both hands and use the electric hedger and the electric weed eater. This may not sound like much, but to someone who lost the use of their arms for a considerable amount of time, it is wonderful to do these functions again. I still cannot lift a stack of dishes like I used to and lift them all together into the cabinet, and I still struggle with opening the lids on jars and other tasks that require a substantial amount of arm strength, but I'm okay with all of that. Why? Because I still have both arms and hands at my side, and when I'm tired and they hurt, I take a rest. What I do know is if I had not taken my physical therapy exercises and strength-building exercises seriously, I would be in far worse shape than I am today. Working through the pain and receiving the gain is all worth it.

So, no, I'm not twenty-five anymore, and I have had more injuries and surgeries than I care to be reminded of, but I'm still kicking and doing the best I can with what I have left of me. My spirit returned to me about eighteen months after it disappeared. There was no significant time or event that caused it to return as far as I can remember. Maybe it was when I began to see progress in doing my physical therapy treatments and I was graduating from one level to another, regaining strength in my left arm. Maybe it was when I was beginning to regain most of my independence again, cooking meals and driving a car again, or just being able to go out on my own again without the use of a walking cane. I really cannot say what driving force made it happen, but I'm just happy it returned to me.

It has been three years and four months since the accident. Not a day goes by that I do not experience some level of pain in my left arm. Many times it feels like a large, hard ball where the plate and screws are. I try not to dwell on it and keep moving forward. When the weather is damp and cold, I do have to put on a sweater or it will go straight to my arm and chill me. Or sometimes I will put on a cotton sleeve over my left arm so that it will be warmer and not hurt so much. Once you get used to taking care of special needs, it is not such a big deal.

In conclusion, my husband and I have a deeper respect for each other now that we have survived a deadly crash. We no longer argue or bicker with each other. Most times when we disagree, we speak our piece and get over it. We say I love you more often at night before we go to sleep. We have a great respect for the highways, freeways, and other cars that cross our paths. We each know the value of having each other in our lives and how it can be lost in an instant. Each time we pass the large wooden cross that represents the man who lost his life that night, we are silent and know it could have been one of us who died.

On August 6, 2011, Jean-Pierre and I celebrated our thirtieth wedding anniversary by renewing our vows in church. I had always wanted to get married in church, but the first time we were married, it was on a party yacht in the Bay Area by Horn Blowers Party Yachts. We cruised around the waters of the San Francisco Bay with seventy-five family members and friends. Celebrating our thirtieth wedding anniversary was special to me because of all we had gone through in life's twists and turns. I turned one day to Jean-Pierre as he was quietly watching television and said to him, "Well after thirty years, do you think I'm worthy of getting married in church?" Without any hesitation, he said, "Yes." I was so thrilled. I began to make arrangements right away, and on that day, my dreams were answered. We had a wonderful priest, Father John Cantwell from St. James Church in Georgetown, California, perform the marriage ceremony, and all our family and friends were present. It was one of the happiest moments in my life as God blessed our marriage.

I have written this book for the suddenly disabled and for the care providers of the suddenly disabled. For additional information, I have added a helpful guide to assist in the enormous task of getting well again and the journey needed to regain independence.

## Listen to the Song of Life

> *Listen to the Song of Life.*
> —*Katharine Hepburn*

On May 1, 2012, I took a break from writing my story and the advice I wanted to provide to others and walked outside and enjoyed the beautiful warm weather. As I gazed at the beautiful, colorful irises in full bloom—white, golden, purple, lavender, and deep blue—I remembered planting them several years ago prior to the accident, and I could see the wonder of life. The gladiolus were beginning to appear in the garden with their sharp pointy tips peeking out of the soil, and all the other beautiful flowers of Mother Nature were beginning to say hello to me. I welcomed the birds flying overhead and the warm sun on my back. I thanked God once again for giving me a second chance at life. I hope I do not disappoint him because I want to give back all that I have gained from the experience of surviving a head-on accident. I hope I have inspired others who suffer from a sudden disability to never give up and hope for a brighter day filled with sunshine.

# Appendix A—Tips for a Successful Recovery

## The Value of a Quality Hospital

A quality hospital is vital for your recovery and care. We were provided with a booklet explaining everything about our hospital stay. As a patient, you have rights, and all hospitals have the responsibility of informing you of the following:

- Patient rights
- Patient safety
- Your hospital stay
- When you arrive
- During your stay
- Patient services
- Before you go home
- If you are being transferred
- A meeting with a discharge planner
- If not being transferred to another facility, home care instructions

When it is time to leave the hospital, the discharge planner in every hospital has the responsibility to inform you and your family members of all you need to know about the facility to which you will be transferred.

During your hospital stay, you should be treated with total dignity and respect. Professionalism and a caring attitude by the employees and the hospital staff are vital. Respect for the patient is a must when providing any service or care. I have found that Kaiser Permanente Medical Centers have always provided quality care and shown professionalism to me. Interpreter services are to be provided to those whose English is a second language. Sign language should also be provided for the hearing impaired.

Unfortunately, I did have some unpleasant experiences in another hospital in which we were placed prior to being admitted to Kaiser Permanente Roseville Medical Center. It was difficult to get hospital staff to answer their call light. Hospital personnel walked past my room and ignored my calls for assistance, and when they did come to my room, I felt they did not have genuine interest in my care and special needs. This was extremely difficult for me to endure during a very painful and emotional time in my life. Therefore, I was ready to be transferred to familiar grounds and admitted to a Kaiser Permanente medical center where I knew I would be cared for in the proper manner.

## Selecting the Right Medical Doctor for You

It is one thing to be assigned a medical doctor for one visit or for just a few visits, but it is another thing to be assigned a medical doctor who will follow your recovery and assign your care and treatment for the long term. Finding and selecting a medical doctor who meets your needs and expectations is vital to your care and recovery. A good physician will not only have a qualified medical degree, have passed the state boards, and have received training at a reputable university or hospital, but he or she should also have a good bedside manner. He or she should be a good listener and care about you as an individual. You should not be treated as a number or a hand or a leg. Bedside manner is important to create a good, trusting relationship between physician and patient. The patient has to feel comfortable with the person who will perform their surgery and confident that the physician will do their absolute best.

Unfortunately, there may be times you will not be able to select your surgeon due to the emergency of your injury, and then we can only hope the right doctor was selected for your surgery. I have worked for over forty years with medical doctors on a daily basis, and like everything else, there are all kinds of personalities and behaviors in every walk of life. Some think they are always right, and others have a caring and listening manner that will melt your heart. In any regards, the medical doctor is to be respected for his wisdom, knowledge, and education, and it is a two-way street of communication between the patient and the physician when working out a relationship that works for both of you. Do not forget it is perfectly fine to ask for a second opinion or to request another doctor for your care if you find that someone is not a good match for you.

## The Importance of Following the Doctor's Orders
I cannot express enough the importance of following doctor's orders during your recovery time. We put a lot of expectations on doctors and little on ourselves to do the work that is necessary to regain our health and physical abilities. The doctors have the training, wisdom, and knowledge to lead us in the right direction, but in the end, it is up to us if we want a full or as full a recovery as possible. Listen to your doctor. Make sure to follow his instructions and to keep all follow-up and return appointments

with your doctor. If you do not improve, call your doctor, if you feel worse, go to the emergency department.

## The Value of Family and Friends

Family and friends are the lifeline to your feeling like yourself again. Even though you may have lost some of your independence when experiencing an sudden disability, family and friends can help you feel connected again in this big wide world of "what's in it for me." Friends and family members are the angels here on earth who help you in any way they can to make your life more comfortable and as stress-free as possible. They are the ones who are willing to prepare your meals, open your mail, write the checks to pay the bills, apply the ice packs on your injuries, get your pain medication with a glass of water, clean your house, drive you to your medical appointments, and assist with any other need you will not be able to take care of on your own. They send an unspoken message of love to you whether you are miserable and behaving in a difficult way due to pain and suffering, or angry your independence has been removed from you, or you are crying your heart out from frustration. Friends and family members are the ones who are there for you and will stand by you through the thick and the thin of your recovery period. Remember to thank them and tell them how special they are to you. Here are some ways our family and friends helped us during our recovery period:

- Stayed overnight at the hospital in our room with us
- Drove us to medical and physical therapy appointments
- Prepared meals for us
- Cut our meat on our plate
- Bought groceries for us
- Wrote our personal checks for us

- Cleaned house for us
- Mailed packages for us
- Took care of our pet
- Helped me get dressed and undressed
- Washed my hair
- Put my jewelry on

## Keeping a Journal of Your Progress and Recovery

Keeping a journal of all progress, activities, and medications is an ideal way to keep track of your recovery period. We noted all the progress and setbacks, such as when my husband had the hiccups and they would not go away, or when he was given some pain medication that had an adverse side effect. In addition, we listed all friends and family members who came by to visit and wish him well.

I think noting the progress of the patient is a positive thing because then one can reflect later how things have improved. Journaling allows for the family members to have hope that in time things will improve. It is also very helpful for the care provider to write their own feelings down and have a place to note what they are experiencing while all this is happening. One of the passages in my husband's journal states how good he looked and how comfortable he was when it was decided that they would cut all his hair off and his beard due to profuse sweating and being in bed all the time. When his hair was completely gone, he said he looked like a convict, and he and the person who did it shared a laugh together.

Another passage in the journal states how his daughter felt when my husband and I met each other after weeks of not seeing each other. She expressed the love we shared between each other with only our eyes since we were both unable to get up out of our wheelchairs and hug each other. It is for all these reasons I believe journaling about the patient's progress and events during the time of recovery is an excellent idea, not only for the patient, but for the care provider as well.

## The Importance of Letter Writing

It's important to get your word out to the ones you love. Letter writing is not only comforting to the receiver, but to the sender as well. Even if you are bedridden, letter writing is a wonderful way to say in your own handwriting, "I care about you, I miss you, and I love you." Computers, cell phones, and texting are all the rage these days, but nothing hits home like a letter in your own handwriting to tell someone you care and that you are thinking about them. To this day, I love sending cards and letters. Let that special someone know you care and then sign it in your own personal signature. Sending a letter of love is good for the soul.

## Selecting a Quality Rehabilitation Center

In my opinion, this is one of the most important decisions your physician and you can agree on—selecting the right rehabilitation center for your recovery. I was very fortunate that my doctor cared about what type of rehab center was right for me and what center would be the best for my recovery process. There are benefits to getting admitted to a top rehab center. The following is a list of services the rehab center I was transferred to offered:

- Dental services
- Vision services
- Hearing services
- Podiatry services
- Psychological services
- Beauty and barber services
- Chaplain services

A top rehab center also offers social workers to provide assistance with the following services:

- Advance directives
- Hospice services
- Financial resources
- Health education materials
- Community resources
- Caregiver support groups
- Transportation services
- Theft and loss reporting
- Clothing services

My rehab center also provided us with "Your Resident's Rights," a handout that is a brief overview of the California Code of Regulations, Title 22. In addition, I received the California Department of Health Services brochure, which explains your right to make healthcare decisions and how you can plan now for your medical care if you are unable to speak for yourself in the future. This information is a requirement of the federal government.

## Transferring to Someone Else's Home for Recovery

First of all, be thankful that someone else has taken on the task of providing your care and the responsibility for your well-being. It is difficult for the person you move in with to have their entire life turn upside down. The house they call their home is now being shared, even if on a temporary basis, and their living space and their privacy has now dwindled.

If you are the care provider, make sure arrangements have been made if needed for a hospital bed to be placed in the home, and that the patient has enough changes of clothes and bedclothes for their stay with you. Watching television can be problematic if the large hospital bed is placed in the middle of the living room, which is usually the largest room in the house. Therefore, television stations have to be shared, and many times, if the patient tires easily, they may want to go to sleep earlier than expected. Meal planning is another aspect to think about because in most cases, the patient is unable to purchase or prepare for their meals, so food must be prepared and readily available for the patient's needs. Medication reminders are a must to make sure the patient is taking their meds on a timely basis. Transportation is almost always needed in order to deliver the patient to and from their medical appointments.

Your temporary new home may have pets you are not used to. At my son's house, he has a cat, and the cat made sure to let me know he was not happy about me moving in and taking his warm, sunny napping spot over with my hospital bed. I'm not a cat lover and tried to make friends with him, but he was not up to it.

Although my son and my granddaughters were excellent in making me feel welcomed and wanted in their home, I know it must have been a big relief when I was ready and able to move back into my home again. Their home could return to normal again. I'm sure the cat was happy I was gone too.

# Appendix B—Helpful Hints for Regaining Independence

The following is a list of hospital supplies and products I used to regain my independence. The proper use of these hospital supplies will help you to transfer from one stage of your healing to another in the recovery process. Some of you will always need the assistance, as I do, of a cane to help with balance, durability, stability, and endurance when traveling, walking long distances, and walking on uneven surfaces. I have grown to be very comfortable with the use of my canes and realize they are now a part of my independence and ability to get around on my own. The following is a full explanation of each hospital supply item and the value they each serve for our comfort and needs.

## Mobility Walking Products

Mobility walking products are wonderful to regain a sense of independence, but people's reaction to you in public may leave a lot to be desired.

*Wheelchairs*

When you are bedridden, a wheelchair can become your new best friend. Why? Regaining your independence is so important to feel whole again. Wheelchairs are not the most comfortable chairs, but they do get you from point A to point B. Many times when you first begin to use a wheelchair, you do not have the full-body strength to wheel yourself around. Here again, you have to depend on others to help out, but soon you can get the hang of it and learn to pull your own weight. Hard floor surfaces are much easier to pull yourself around on. Carpets have a tendency to slow you down, and it can become difficult to maneuver your wheelchair.

I recall a particular incident when I was just recovering from foot surgery and my husband was wheeling me around Old Sacramento to attend his work Christmas party. Even my own husband grew tired of wheeling me around on the old wooden boardwalk. The uneven boards on the walk were causing the wheelchair to bounce unevenly, and I began to feel like an old sack of potatoes. I remember being thrown about by my husband pushing me and trying to get my large body over the uneven and cracked boards. I wanted to just shrink up and fly away. I was so angry with him, thinking he was being inconsiderate, but now looking back, maybe he had to place that amount of pressure just to get my big body over the wooden boards! In any event, I was all dressed up and just wanted to die.

It was interesting using a wheelchair out in public while grocery shopping at Costco. I was getting stares at folks when I was in their aisle and they had to move around me. Their looks of hatred said, "What are you doing in my aisle?" However, when using a wheelchair in the rehab center, I was able to get up whenever I wanted, whether it was three in the morning or not. When I got strong enough, I would use my wheelchair as a walker to get me from my bed to the grand lobby. The nursing staff frowned on this type of use of my wheelchair, but it made me feel more independent to use it as a walker, and when I was tired, I would sit in it and wheel myself back to my room.

When my husband arrived at the rehab center, we were both in wheelchairs, and I dubbed us the Wheelchair Brigade. It was a way to add some humor to the fact that we were now both in wheelchairs instead of walking side by side as we had done for so many years.

*Walkers*

I did not use a walker during my recovery period, but my husband used a walker when he came home to recover. The walker is very useful for gaining your balance and stability, and it also assures you that you have something to hold on to if you should tire easily. The walker makes you feel like you have graduated from sitting in a wheelchair to being upright and standing on your own two feet again, which is a real accomplishment when you've been in a wheelchair for some time. For those people who have to depend on a walker permanently, there are several different styles to choose from. Some walkers come with seats and baskets so that you can sit and carry different items when in use.

*Hemi Walker Canes*

A Hemi Walker is a cane that looks similar to a small stepladder. It is shaped like a ladder and bridges out to add balance to your walking. It is a heavy cane, and you are unable to go anywhere quickly. In my opinion, it is made to add stability and balance to your walking and to prevent falling with the additional ability to stop when you need to and to lean on it to rest. When I graduated from a wheelchair, I was given a Hemi Walker cane in the rehab center. Using a Hemi Walker cane was another step in the right direction of gaining more independence for me. It enabled me to stand upright and on my own two legs. There is a great sense of independence when you can once again stand on your own.

## Four-Prong Cane

A four-prong cane is another cane to slow down your walking and to assist you with stability and balance. Again, it is impossible to walk fast with it, but as my physical therapists stated, "It is not always best to go fast." As for me, fast was always a part of my life, but I have to say when a sudden disability happens fast, it not part of your vocabulary. Slow and easy wins the race. Having safety, stability, security, and a sense of balance is the best you can hope for when healing and recovering. As I age, fast is no longer part of my everyday life. When I try to rush, I usually end up hurting myself or getting out of breath.

## Standard Walking Canes

All canes are adjustable for different heights and for right- and left-hand users. Once you graduate to a standard walking cane, you come to respect it as an old friend and know the value of it. To have the use of a cane at your side to assist you when the walking gets tough is a much-needed reassurance. I have respect for all my canes. I even keep the four-prong cane in my laundry-room closet for safekeeping.

One of my challenges when first using a cane was to walk with two canes at the same time. It is somewhat like skiing on land. It was very difficult to get used to, and I was really challenged by having to learn to master it. My first time using it, my husband parked our newly purchased truck in a small parking mall, and I got out to go to the bakery across the way. I was trying very hard to learn how to walk with two canes and was going rather slowly while crossing the intersection when I heard a loud voice from a male teenager yell to me from a car window, "Lady, why don't you learn to walk first!" I was so humiliated that when I reached my husband standing near his truck, I burst into tears. At that point, life seemed so cruel, and I had come such a long way, but no one cared or knew. It was such a humbling experience for me; I had always been so independent.

*Tie-Up Fabric Braces*
Since I'm a fall risk and we like to travel, which requires a lot of walking, I have used tie-up fabric braces to support my feet and ankles. This has helped tremendously in sustaining my balance and has allowed me to walk much farther when tired. We went to Greece, our second trip there. On the first trip, I missed seeing the Parthenon way up on the hillside due to my instability and poor balance. I chose to sit down below on a bench as my husband climbed the steep hill to the site. The second time we went to Greece, I was determined to see the Parthenon firsthand and not through the lenses of a camera. I was determined to make it on my own with the help of a cane and the tie-up fabric ankle braces. I made it, but I was so tired by the time I reached the site I could not truly catch all the wonderful things to see. But I had made it, and that in itself was quite an accomplishment.

## Other Items for Building Your Independence
Once at my son's home, the physical therapist recommended that I purchase some items that would increase my independence and help lift my spirit. The following are some of the items I purchased online to assist me with everyday living:

*Elastic Shoestrings*
They're inexpensive and have lots of benefits. Elastic shoestrings allow you to put your shoes on without having to tie them and

without having to lean over to put them on and take them off. Your shoes stay tied, and you just push your shoes off and slip into them when ready to use them. The elastic shoe strings never have to be tied but once.

## Wooden One-Arm Cutting Board

This item is essential when working in the kitchen and trying to prepare dinner on your own again. It is a wooden board with a nail right in the center of it to hold the piece of meat or vegetable for stabilization while cutting it into smaller pieces. Once I got the hang of this cutting board, it was love at first sight. I no longer had to ask anyone to help me out in the kitchen when it came to cutting.

## Pedal Exerciser

This is a helpful way to achieve exercise for your legs when you are unable to stand for long periods. The pedal exerciser is used while you are in a sitting position and provides a good workout for improving the strength in both your legs without the difficulty of losing your balance while standing. I enjoyed this piece of exercise equipment, and it was actually fun to use.

## The Full-Page Magnifier

It was very useful, particularly because I was without eyeglasses for a few weeks. My glasses were broken in the accident. I prefer the full-page magnifier over the smaller handheld magnifying glass because you can place the full-page magnifier directly over an article to read it in full without having to move the smaller one over the paragraphs.

## Shower Chair

Use a shower chair when you are too weak or unstable to stand alone, or even with assistance from a care provider. It allows you to sit for however much time it takes to wash yourself and take care of your daily needs. It is made of a stable white plastic, is easy to clean, and has a wide seat for comfort. There are large suction cups on the chair's legs, so you can feel safe from slipping or sliding in a wet tub. The shower chair has adjustable legs for increasing and decreasing leg heights.

## Moving Carts with Wheels

I learned to use a cart with wheels to move my clean laundry from one room to the other. The carts are valuable for moving any item, such as food trays from the kitchen to your TV trays in the family room. I have even used the office chair, which has easy movable wheels, to transport files from one room to the next.

## MCR Lightweight Reacher or "The Grabber"

I had seen these handy little items in *Harriet Carter* magazines and other discount magazines that you find in your mailbox. I would look at the description and think, *Sure it does all those things.* However, the grabber is a lifesaver for those of us who are too short or unable to reach for items that fall on the floor or into the washing machine, such as a piece of paper or a coin. The grabber actually works and works very well at that. It can reach for many items that are over your head and out of reach like the toilet paper and paper towel rolls that someone in the house put on the top shelf. There is a magnet at the end of the grabber that will pick up small iron or steel objects. The grabber has never failed me, and I swear by it, so the next time you need help reaching for an item, remember the grabber. It will be another friend for life. I have actually found myself searching around the house for it in such a fury like I had lost something valuable and had to find it. The grabber is with me for life!

## Clothing: Dressing with One Arm

I found that most of my clothes were not made for people with the use of only one arm, and putting on jewelry like necklaces and earrings was impossible. I started to look for clothes I had in my closet that had snaps instead of buttons, and pants that had elastic waistbands. I had some dusters or house coats and a few pairs of jogging pants with elastic waistbands. I would recommend these types of clothing for anyone who has difficulty getting dressed each day. Jogging style jackets or tops that had a zipper in the front or snaps were also much easier for me to handle on my own. Combing my hair was the worst for me because my husband was not gifted in fixing it in a style I was comfortable with, so I became very frustrated knowing I could not style my own hair.

## Being Prepared for the Unexpected

Post-traumatic stress disorder (PTSD) is something I have learned to live with and to work on every day to help myself live a full life. There is not a lot known about this disorder, but it is something that can haunt those who have it every day of their lives. Like most disorders, it is as unique and individualized as the person who has been diagnosed with PTSD.

The following is a condensed version of an article from MedicineNet.com.

"Disaster Survivors Face PTSD Risk"

Medical Author: Melissa Conrad Stoppler, MD
Medical Editor: William C. Shiel, Jr. MD, FCAP, FACR

Post-traumatic stress order (PTSD) is a psychiatric condition that can develop following any traumatic, catastrophic life experience. PTSD symptoms vary among individuals and also vary in severity from mild to disabling. PTSD symptoms can include one or more of the following:

- Flashbacks about the traumatic event
- Feelings of estrangement or detachment
- Nightmares
- Sleep disturbances
- Impaired functioning
- Occupational instability
- Memory disturbances
- Family discord
- Parenting or martial difficulties

The following is a list of the unexpected experiences you might have. It helps to be aware and to expect the unexpected.

- Easily tired
- Sleepier than usual
- Experiencing more pain than you thought
- Uncomfortable most of time
- Angry and frustrated with your situation
- May need to be put in diapers temporarily
- May need assistance with showering or bathing
- May need someone else to tie your shoes
- May take longer than expected to recover or heal
- May need more surgeries
- May need help getting in and out of bed
- May find yourself alone at times taking care of yourself

## Pathways to Get Through the Recovery Period

Here are a few suggestions to help you get through the recovery period:

## Well Writing

*Well Writing for Health after Trauma and Abuse,* by Ellen H. Taliaferro, MD, is a book about five Well Writing ways to regain your health and life. Before the accident, I actually went to Dr. Taliaferro's writing workshops and purchased this book. I found it to be an even greater asset after the accident. Although the book focuses on domestic violence, I discovered that the techniques also apply to overcoming pain and illness, reducing stress, recognizing negative emotions, and taking action from wherever you are. It is a book about being a survivor.

## Art Therapy

I for one have always enjoyed artwork and different media, such as oil, ink and pen, pencil, chalk, and acrylics. However, I do not always have the time to think about giving myself this pleasure to do some artwork. I have found through artwork one can become totally absorbed in the process of producing a piece of art that is truly yours alone. When you put full concentration into your artwork, you will discover the pain is not as great, and the discomfort seems to go away. If only for a while, there is a sense of relief. It is also like reading because of the concentration level and the quiet time it generates. However, you are producing a product that you can be proud of, and it has your unique touch to it.

## Pet Therapy

In a hospital or a rehab center, pet-therapy organizations are a wonderful way to lift your spirits. These highly trained dogs are a comfort to all who come in contact with them. They allow you to pet them or just sit quietly with them and enjoy their company. At home, having your own pet at your side is another wonderful comfort. Your pet may have missed you during your absence and may want to stay nearby to make sure you do not leave again. The love they possess and the desire to care for you and comfort you is immeasurable. Once you are well enough to take your pet for a walk or to teach him or her new tricks, it can be another rewarding experience. Just knowing your pet is by your side and ready to provide you with love and licks is a great reward in itself. Taking time to be with a pet warms the heart and comforts the soul.

*Aromatherapy*

This is one area that is often overlooked but can add a relaxing feeling to your environment. Lighting aroma candles, burning incense, or the aroma from a beautiful flower arrangement can lift anyone's spirit. Just boiling some cinnamon sticks in a pot of water adds a wonderful aroma in the kitchen and family room areas. Adding scents of lavender, coconut, or bath salts to the tub is another wonderful way aromatherapy works on the mind and comforts the soul. Soft, relaxing music with the lights turned down low can relax your mind and comfort you. Add a warm blanket during the winter or a cool compress on your forehead during the hot days of summer; this can be another delight.

*Swimming*

Taking a dip in the swimming pool or swimming hole is a wonderful way to relax your aching muscles. I have used a swimming pool with my left arm broken and in a sling and with a torn knee on my right leg. Yes, I hobbled along, but there were times I tried my hand at swimming a stroke or two. The water allows you to become weightless, and what would cause pain out of the water is usually minimized once submerged in the water. Once I was able to be well enough to go swimming, I enjoyed it immensely. I purchased swimming gloves, which are webbed at the fingers, to help build strength in my arms and hands. Working with swimming gloves under water helps build up the tolerance against the water, which in turn helps strengthen the muscles in your arms and hands. By the end of summer, I was swimming one thousand strokes with both arms in one half hour. Another benefit of swimming is you are pretty much using every muscle in your body at once. Therefore, in a short time, you can see the results of losing inches from your body, and you begin to look great.

After a good swim, I have always felt refreshed. There were times when my arms and hands would ache from pushing them to the limit, but it was a good pain for a change. It allowed me the time to work at building my strength and nurturing my heart as I was trying my best to become whole again

*Chronic Pain Management Classes*
In these classes, you learn breathing and relaxation techniques, such as Pilates, and the goal is to maintain a healthy lifestyle. Tai Chi is another class you can take that promotes good health, peace of mind, coordination, and balance between the body and the mind.

## What You Need to Move Back Home
Coming home from the hospital or the rehab center is a joyous day. However, you must be prepared and ready to return home and somewhat take care of yourself. There is no 24/7 nursing staff, and there is no one there to wake you up in the middle of the night to give you your pain medication or to take your vital signs. You are pretty much on your own unless you have made arrangements for someone to be there or you have prepared a well-managed self-care program to help you through the difficult times of healing and the recovery process.

The following is a list of supplies and items we had ready and available for returning home:

- A hospital bed was placed in our living room for my husband. We converted the space into a hospital room for his needs and comfort.
- There was a wheelchair and a walker for him to get around the house.
- We moved all furniture out of the way of his traveling path.
- At his bedside were extra pillows, blankets, a urinal on the bed rail, and near his bed was a TV table with tissues, a water pitcher with lid, a glass, his cell phone to schedule pain medication reminders, and medications.
- Placed behind his hospital bed was our dining-room table converted into a hospital supply unit.
- We placed a change of clothes, bedclothes, all other items that one may need for surgical wound care, cleaning items, and things that are needed for his comfort and care so that we wouldn't have to search the house for these items.
- A journal or log book to write down any concerns or issues to discuss with the doctor, a large plastic wash basin, towels, toothpaste, toothbrush, blood pressure monitor, thermometer, and oximeter to measure blood oxygen levels are also helpful to have.
- Anything the patient will need on a daily basis was placed on the large table for quick use and readiness.
- The oxygen tank machine and two extra oxygen tanks were placed next to his bedside. An instruction manual for all hospital equipment was also placed on the large table for quick access.

# Hospital Supply Equipment You May Need at Home

*Blood Pressure Cuff and Pulse Monitor*
A blood pressure cuff and pulse monitor can be purchased at most pharmaceutical stores. They are fairly inexpensive and easy to use and will monitor your vitals with accuracy.

*Oxygen Cylinder and Concentrator Systems*
A manual for the Oxygen Cylinder and Concentrator Systems was given to us when we received our oxygen machine and additional oxygen tanks. The representative of the oxygen company provided a demonstration and went over the checklist.

*Patient Instructions for Oxygen Cylinder and Concentrator Systems,* by Apria Healthcare, is a very thorough booklet the representative will go over with you. The checklist includes the following:

Demonstrate the following:

- How to turn machine on
- How to set flow rate
- Alarm function
- How to clean filter
- How to care for cabinet
- If required, how to fill and attach humidifier bottle
- If required, how to assemble and disassemble humidifier bottle
- If required, how to clean the humidifier bottle
- Have patient/ caregiver demonstrate all of the above

Safety Information:

- Explain oxygen safety precautions
- Post "No Smoking" signs
- Explain need for grounded outlet
- Explain importance of following cleaning procedure
- Explain proper procedure during power failure
- Explain Apria Healthcare's equipment delivery and maintenance schedule
- Explain Oxygen Concentrator section
- Give patient/caregiver Apria Healthcare's telephone number to call for routine and after-hours equipment problems
- Explain how to obtain help if a medical emergency arises

There is detailed information in the booklet about many other pertinent things regarding oxygen use and safety, such as travel tips, care of your oxygen tubing, and oxygen concentrator troubleshooting.

*Oximeter*

In addition to having to administer oxygen for my husband, we also had to use an oximeter to record and measure his blood oxygen levels. Many times his hands and fingers were especially cold, and we had to warm them up before getting an accurate oximeter reading.

The oximeter we purchased was CMS Model 50-DL Pulse Finger Oximeter. It is easy to read, and the cost was approximately $90.95. We purchased this product from Southeastern Medical Supply, Inc. (httpp://www.semedicalsupply.com/cms-50dl.htm).

## How to Request Home Care Services

The method I use to request home care services was to make an appointment with my husband's doctor and clearly explain all the things we were not able to do by ourselves. Once we met with the doctor, I prepared a typed list stating all the reasons we were in need of home care services for our safety. A typed list is a form of documentation requesting home care services, and it should be placed in your medical record that you are requesting these services. Keep a copy for your own files.

## What to Look for When Requesting a Home Care Service

Once we returned home for from the rehab center, we realized we would need additional assistance with our daily activities and to continue our wound care and physical therapy sessions. We were fortunate to have wonderful, professional home care services. Here are some helpful hints when selecting a quality home care service.

Find a quality and professional home care service that is located close to your home. It is not only convenient, but most often the care provider will be on time for your scheduled appointments and not caught up in traffic jams and other details.

All top home care services will provide brochure information on all the services they provide, and it is helpful to select a home care service that covers the majority of services you will need, such as physical therapists, occupational therapists, speech therapists, registered nurses, medical social workers, and certified health aides.

It is equally important to have friendly and professional staff members who are willing to listen to your needs, issues, and concerns, and they should be able to answer your questions. If they are not able to answer your questions, then they should be able to lead you in the right direction so that your questions will be answered or follow up with you in a timely manner with answers to your questions. Building a friendship with these health care professionals is essential in your recovery and healing process. If they are not a good fit for you, then you will need to look elsewhere for your home care needs.

A quality home care service will also provide handouts with detailed information on the following topics:

- Infection control and ways to help prevent infections
- Signs and symptoms of infection
- Fall prevention program instructions for the family
- Instructions for measuring pain
- Home safety / fire safety
- Major emergency preparedness tips

They will have available handouts on "red flags"—symptoms and what to look out for if there is profuse sweating, cold, weakness, dizziness, or shortness of breath, as these are areas of concern. They will state what to expect, such as some sweating but not profuse. They will inform you that being dizzy and just sitting down is okay, but dizziness with activity is not okay.

## What to Expect When There Are More Surgeries

The thought of more surgeries is not pleasant. However, if the surgery is to relieve the pain or for corrective reasons, it may very well be worth it in the long run. Rebuilding your body strength after additional surgeries can take more time than expected, but the rewards are well worth it if the surgery is successful. Sometimes you just have to put your faith in someone else's hands and hope and pray for the best result. I was lucky that all my surgeries were for solid reasons and with better results than if I had chosen not to have the surgery. No two surgeries for me were the same in regard to the pain level I experienced or the time in the recovery process. Therefore, the only thing I could rely on was a positive frame of mind and a willingness to sacrifice the pain for the gain of functionality and reduction of pain. When you are faced with additional surgeries, think of it in this way: you have already gone down this road, so plan well for the path ahead while making your recovery process as comfortable as possible, and remember to ask for help. We cannot do everything on our own. Asking for help is not a sign of weakness but a wise decision in the healing process.

## What to Expect during the Recovery Process

As I mentioned, no two surgeries are exactly the same, and the same applies to the recovery process. With some surgeries, you may become more nauseated and feel weaker than you did with the previous surgery. You may or may not experience more pain, and you may or may not have more trouble going to sleep or finding a more comfortable position. Just know that this too will pass and that as you follow your doctors' and physical therapist's orders, the pain will slow down and then dwindle away as you progress with each new day. Work at remaining positive and doing activities that are pleasant for you or relaxing. This will help in dealing with the boredom of being homebound and recovering. Remember to stay social with your friends and to make sure you are exposed to activities that will help pass the time. Just sitting in front of the television and channel surfacing can get old. Try activities that require more mental stimulation.

## Activities for the Homebound

Here is a list of activities for the homebound during your recovery period.

- Card games
- Board games
- Puzzles
- Dominoes
- Reading a good book
- Video games
- Crossword puzzles
- Creating a family tree
- Looking at family photo albums
- Cleaning out old paper files
- Bead making
- Updating your personal address book
- Viewing old home movies
- Closing your eyes and listening to your favorite music
- Writing five affirmations and sticking to them
- Listening to an audiobook
- Tape recording your favorite memories
- Scrapbooking
- Reading old love letters
- Writing a bucket list
- Writing down a list of a hundred things you love to do, and then doing some of them now and planning some for when you recover

## Physical Therapy Exercises

Here is a list of just some of the physical therapy exercises I did each and every day until I regained the strength and mobility in my left arm and right arm. The physical therapy exercises were done multiple times a day, working through the pain for the gain of having both arms' functions return to me. Most of these exercises were provided to us by the Kaiser Permanente Roseville Physical Therapy Department:

*Susan's Beginning Daily Exercises*

- Touch each finger to your thumb
- Massage each finger up toward heart
- Shoulder shrugs
- Arm sliding up and down across chest
- Chicken dance
- Pendulum
- Arm overhead lying down
- No weight on left arm
- Knees to chest right side only and hold one minute
- Back safety: avoid pushing, pulling, lifting more than ten pounds
- Avoid twisting and bending waist
- Log roll in and out of bed

As my health improved, more exercises were suggested. Here is a sample of just a few I did every day, multiple times a day, to regain the function and strength in my left arm:

- The hand physical therapist would massage my hand and wrists each time I would visit her, and then she would use a whirlwind of "crushed cork" in a machine, such as a sand blaster with warm air, to also massage my hand and wrists.
- I was given different color sponge squares to squeeze with my left hand in order to improve my strength.
- Pulley Exercises: Sit in a chair below your pulley setup. The affected arm rests in one handle of the pulley, and the unaffected hand grasps the other handle. With the unaffected arm, pull down on the cord so that the affected arm is raised. Stop when you notice the shoulder blade starting to rise.

- Self-Stretching Activities and Flexion Exercises: These exercises are essential if you want a good recovery, but these in particular can be very painful in the beginning. The good news is as you gradually improve, the pain will subside. Some examples follow.
- Raise arms from sides and lower toward floor above head. Go as far as possible without pain.
- Shoulder Range of Motion Exercise (self-stretching activities): Keep palm of hand against doorframe and elbow bent at ninety degrees. Turn body from fixed hand until a stretch is felt. Hold five seconds. Repeat ten times. Do four sessions per day.
- Shoulder Towel Stretch for Internal Rotation: Pull involved arm up behind back by pulling towel upward (I used my cane) with uninvolved arm. Hold five seconds. Repeat ten times. Do four sessions a day.

Then I graduated to the shoulder-strengthening activities!

- **Shoulder-Strengthening Active Resistive External Rotation**. Using tubing and keeping elbow in at side, rotate arm outward away from body. Be sure to keep forearm parallel to floor. Two sets. Repeat twenty times. Do two sessions per day.
- **Shoulder-Strengthening Active Resistive Internal Rotation.** Using tubing and keeping elbow in at side, rotate arm inward across body. Be sure to keep forearm parallel to floor. Two sets. Repeat twenty times. Do two sessions per day.
- **Shoulder-Strengthening Active Resistive Extension.** Using tubing, pull arm back. Be sure to keep elbow straight. Two sets. Repeat twenty times. Do two sessions per day.

- **Bilateral Scapular Retraction.** Wrap tubing around both fists, and other end of tubing behind a door closed. Pull arms back while bringing shoulder blades together as if rowing a boat. Repeat 20–30 times. Do two sets/sessions. Do 2–3 sessions a day.

My husband had his own physical therapy exercises to do.

**Beginning Daily Leg Exercises**
- Four-pound weight on each leg, one on ankle, and one on bad cut leg placed on foot and wrapped around.
- Raise and extend legs at knee area while sitting in a chair until tired and then measure oxygen level with oximeter.
- Next exercise use same weight. Stand up holding on to walker, left leg at knee length until tired, and then measure oxygen level with oximeter.
- Three times a day.

**Ankle Foot Exercises Resisted Dorsiflexion**
- With tubing anchored in doorjamb, pull foot toward face.
- Return slowly to starting position. Relax.
- Repeat 20–30 times. Do 2–3 sessions per day. Two Sets.

**Cervical Spine Flexibility: Corner Stretch**
- Standing in corner with hands at shoulder level and feet 12 feet from corner, lean forward until a comfortable stretch is felt across chest.
- Hold thirty seconds. Repeat three times. Do 2–3 times per day.

## Creating a Safe Environment

Many accidents begin at home and can be prevented by using helpful techniques to create a safe environment. For the suddenly disabled, there are proper techniques to use when getting in and out of bed and taking a shower or bath. I have noted some helpful instructions our care providers at Accent Home Care Services gave to us.

*Instructions for Getting In Bed*
- On right side of bed, sit back on the bed as far as possible.
- As you lie down, tuck your knees up and place feet on the bed.
- Roll back with your knees bent.

*Instructions for Getting Out of Bed*
- Bend both knees.
- Roll onto your right side.
- Feet over edge, push up with your right arm.

*How to Take a Shower and Do a Bath Transfer*
- Bring wheelchair or walker close to the tub.
- Step into tub with left leg first.
- If you use wheelchair, lock it first before getting up, then push off of chair.
- Use handrail.
- Turn around in bath chair and sit down.
- When done, push up from shower chair.
- Step over tub.
- Sit in wheelchair or use walker to bed area.
- Turn walker in front of you to get out of tub.
- Special note: Place grab bars on right side of bath and back wall.

- Do all important things in the morning.
- Do less important things in the evening.

## Helpful Hints to Avoid Falling and to Stay Safe

*Use Handrails*
One of my worst falls was because I missed the second step on a staircase, and I did not hold on to the handrail. The result was I broke my left arm and tore my right knee. To this day, I will always hold on to the handrail when walking up and down a staircase.

*Avoid Rushing*
Another time I had a terrible fall was when we were rushing to go to a boat party, and I was wearing a pair of sandals. It was very hot, my feet were sweaty, and the sandal went one way, my foot went the other direction, and I fell on the boat dock. The metal ridging of the dock ripped open my wedding-band finger. It was extremely painful.

*Corrective Shoes*
I have learned not to rush anymore, always giving myself enough time to get there safely. I have also purchased shoes that help my balance and help me to walk with comfort and ease. The shoes are not glamorous and are expensive, but they have allowed me to walk much further and without pain when traveling and walking long distances. I have yet to fall when wearing them. As a dress shoe for ladies, selecting a one-inch wedge heel is better for walking comfort and balance distribution, and you will not be in pain at the end of the event. Pumps with a low square heel are also better than any high heel for comfort and balance.

*Safety Alert Necklace*

Another device I have used is a "safety alert" necklace with a chain you wear around your neck. If you should fall, pressing the center button will activate the response rescue teams in the area. Although I have never had to use it, I have felt more secure knowing I'm wearing it when no one else is home and I'm working around the house.

*Carry a Cell Phone*

A close friend also informed me that when she works in the garden or outside, she always brings her cell phone with her and clips it onto her jeans in case of an emergency or fall.

*Reconsider Personal Habits*

These safety guidelines were given to us by Apria Healthcare. The following is a brief outline of the entire contents of this handout:

- When walking, stay alert to unexpected obstacles—cords, furniture, pets, toys, etc.
- Avoid rushing to answer phones or the door.
- Take time to make sure your balance is steady before sitting up or standing.
- Wear shoes that are supportive and snug fitting with low heels and nonslippery soles.
- Don't walk around with only socks on your feet.
- If carrying packages, make sure your view isn't blocked and that you have a hand free for opening doors, holding on to railings, or steadying your balance.
- Keep alert for uneven, broken, or slippery pavement, sidewalks, and ramps.
- Don't rush to cross streets, especially if wet or icy.

- Consider using a cane or walker.
- Find out if your medications might make you feel dizzy, drowsy, or unsteady.
- If you live alone, keep in regular contact with friends, family, or neighbors.

There is more information on this handout regarding looking around your home and considering obstacles inside and outside your home. It also provides information for emergencies and what to do if you fall.

## Celebrate Your Gains and Accomplishments

Do not forget to celebrate you gains and pat yourself on the back for all the good work you have achieved when you have mastered each step of the recovery process. Just like any event, when you tried your best and worked through the pain for the gain, it should be celebrated as a milestone in your recovery period. During your recovery process, you work through the mental, physical, and emotional aspects of healing. Celebrating gives special attention to your achievements and efforts. Here are just a few suggestions for celebrating each step of the way to reaching your personal goal:

- Celebrate with a glass of champagne.
- Have a special dinner with a special someone.
- Enjoy an ice-cream sundae.
- Plan an event to honor and thank all those who have helped you get through your recovery.
- Plan a trip or vacation.
- Buy a delicious, decadent piece of chocolate and let it slowly melt in your mouth.
- Buy a new outfit.
- Purchase a new hat.

- Plan a small party with friends to celebrate.
- Get a massage.
- Get a new hairdo or color.

Celebrate, celebrate, celebrate for just being alive and that there is a tomorrow.

## Learning to Travel with a Disability

Comfort and saving your energy and strength while traveling a long distance are important. Making arrangements with the airport to have airport personnel transport you by wheelchair from point A to point B is essential in today's multibuilding airports and terminals. These employees are responsible for your making your connection on time and safely. It will save your energy, and you will not have to carry your own luggage.

When you are disabled, getting totally exhausted before you arrive at your destination can be avoided. Reducing the weight of your luggage by packing lightly is a benefit. Do you really need a full change of clothes for every day you are traveling? I have found that jewelry and scarves are wonderful accessories for changing the look of an outfit from causal to more formal. Instead of taking the entire travel book with you, tear out only the pages of interests regarding your destination. Remember to pack all needed medications and creams. I never travel without Extra-Strength Tylenol because I want to be prepared for the unexpected migraine or any discomfort from a surgery or arthritic site. These are the essentials for traveling with a disability. They are as important as a good book to read while on the long plane ride. My husband takes an inflatable pillow for the airplane trip to add comfort to his neck and back.

## Better Lifestyle Hints and Milestones for the Suddenly Disabled

- A Jacuzzi bubble bath for those tried muscles
- A swim in the pool for relaxing the spirit, body, and mind
- Completing your physical therapy exercises
- Eating a healthy meal
- Being pain free
- Getting back to normal
- Being around your family
- Celebrating your milestones
- Being with your loved one
- A smile from your grandchild
- Not falling down for one year
- Not having any more corrective surgeries
- Working in your garden again
- Not being afraid to drive your car again
- Having your pet by your side and loving you
- Getting a bouquet of flowers
- Seeing old friends
- A good laugh

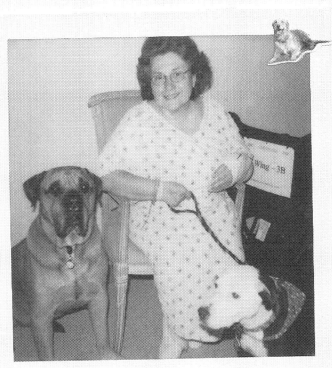

Dino, Susan & Maxie

Eskaton Rehabilitation Center
January 2009
Visiting with pet therapy dogs

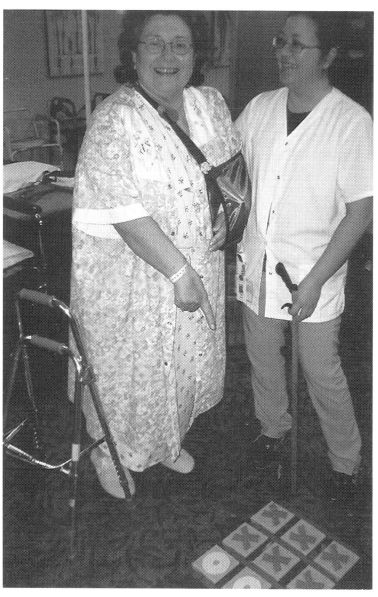

Physical Therapy Department, January 2009
Winning at tic-tac-toe!
The physical therapist is holding the grabber,
and I am using the Hemi Walker cane.

# A Celebration of Life

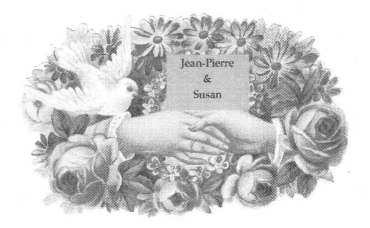

Jean-Pierre
&
Susan

An invitation to a Celebration of Life,
a "thank-you" reception for all your excellent care and in
celebrating God's gift for a new life on April 26, 2009

# A Celebration of Life
## and
# Thank You Reception
### *Event Program*


1:00 pm Socializing Reception

2:00pm Welcome and Thank You
Rescue Team, Health Care Professionals,
Family and Friends

Recognition of Special People
Cool Fire Department
Georgetown Fire Department
1st Lady on the Scene

Unveiling of Oil Painting by Jean-Pierre
Special Recipients

"Make A Wish" Balloons Toss!

Program Event flyer placed inside Celebration of Life invitation

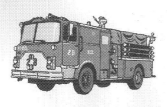

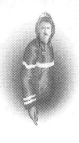

# Cool Fire Department
# &
# Georgetown Fire Department

# Thank YOU!
# for
# "Saving Our Lives"

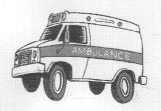

Thank-you flyer placed on story board
at Celebration of Life event

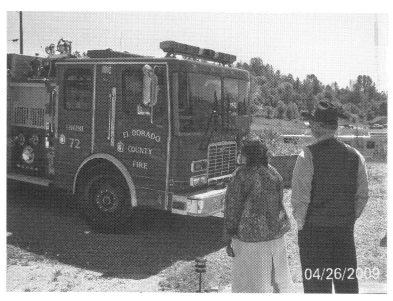

The Georgetown fire truck arriving to our
"Celebration of Life" event to thank the firemen for
our rescue. Foreground: Jean-Pierre and me.

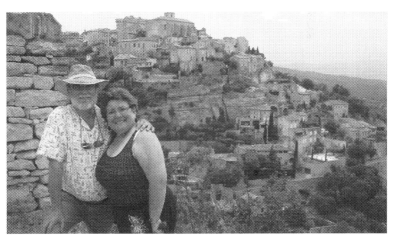

May 2010 Southern France trip
(Note scar on my left arm from surgery in November 2009)

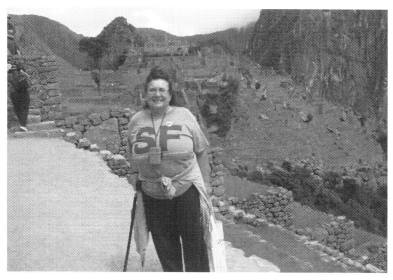

I made it! Machu Picchu, Peru
December 4, 2011

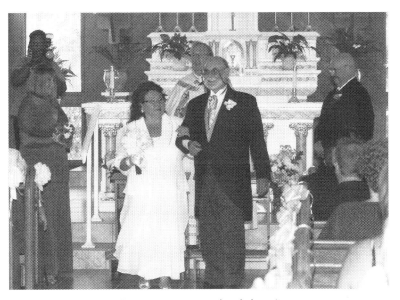

Renewing our vows and celebrating our
thirtieth wedding anniversary
August 6, 2011

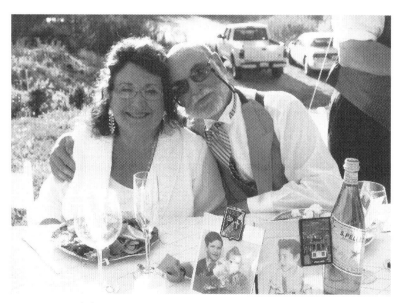

Celebrating our thirtieth wedding anniversary